Clinical Cases

Clinical Cases

A Step-by-Step Approach

Andrew Solomon, BM BCH MA(Hons) DM FRCP
Consultant Physician
East and North Hertfordshire NHS Trust
Stevenage, UK

Julia Anstey, BSc (Hons) MBBS
Foundation Doctor
Somerset NHS Foundation Trust
Taunton, UK

Liora Wittner, MBBS BSc
Resident in Internal Medicine
Shamir Medical Centre
Be'er Ya'akov, Israel

With contributions from
Priti Dutta, MBBS BSc FRCR
Consultant Radiologist
Royal Free London NHS Foundation Trust
London, UK

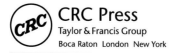

CRC Press
Taylor & Francis Group
Boca Raton London New York

CRC Press is an imprint of the
Taylor & Francis Group, an **informa** business

First edition published 2021
by CRC Press
6000 Broken Sound Parkway NW, Suite 300, Boca Raton, FL 33487-2742

and by CRC Press
2 Park Square, Milton Park, Abingdon, Oxon, OX14 4RN

ISBN: 978-0-8153-6728-4 (hbk)
ISBN: 978-0-8153-6714-7 (pbk)
ISBN: 978-1-351-25772-5 (ebk)

DOI: 10.1201/9781351257725

Typeset in Minion Pro
by Deanta Global Publishing Services, Chennai, India

Contents

Foreword

When Aneurin Bevan set up the NHS in 1948, medicine was dominated by relatively acute illness. Pneumonia, industrial accidents, childhood infections and the like were the order of the day. This cultural legacy lasted well into the modern era with many textbooks and much medical education still focusing disproportionately on the acute illness. Much of my own post-graduate pedagogic experience was dominated by clinical case books teasing the learner with the differential diagnosis of acute hepatitis, lengthy lists of rare causes of pericarditis, photosensitive rashes and orogenital ulceration. The plain truth of the matter is that the majority of the time, medicine isn't really like this any longer. We have long since transitioned to the era of the long-term condition, the chronic illness and the poly-comorbid patient. Patients and their diseases frequently coexist, side by side, for decades, the one influencing the course of the other and vice versa.

With this enlightening, educational, insightful and sensitively written series of cases, the clinical case book is brought into the modern era. The authors have pulled off a masterful job of interweaving contemporary medical education, updating the reader on the latest guidance and thinking, with a sensitive and at times touching investigation of the effect of patients' diseases on their life course and vice versa. Students, graduates preparing for specialist exams and others will enjoy and benefit from this lovely book.

Professor Jeremy Turner, MBBS BSc FRCP DPhil (Oxon)
Consultant Endocrinologist
Department of Diabetes & Endocrinology
NNUH

Honorary Professor
Norwich Medical School

Clinical Director
NIHR CRN: Eastern Research Network

Foreword

A consultation is a meeting of two experts: the doctor who is an expert in medicine and the person accessing care who is an expert in how their condition affects them and their life. As the National Education Lead for Realistic Medicine at NHS Education for Scotland, I am passionate in supporting newly and nearly qualified doctors to adopt a person-centred approach to their work, which may sometimes look and feel quite different from the style of their more senior colleagues.

People with a serious or chronic health condition live with the implications of it every day. As a doctor, your interactions form only a tiny part of the lived experience of the people who seek your help. I would suggest that for your medical advice and intervention to have any impact, you need to know what matters to the person who will live with the consequences. Shared decision-making, where people are fully involved in the healthcare decisions that affect their lives, should be the standard consultation style in 21st-century medicine.

This book provides a novel approach to understanding the trajectory of disease processes over time. But more than that, this book demonstrates how the wishes and goals of the person at the centre shape the decisions made and the outcomes.

Take the case of Mrs Deane, the 76-year-old woman who is diagnosed with metastatic breast cancer. A different person may have chosen to try chemotherapy, but Mrs Deane is clear that this is not the route for her. This is a reasonable decision; just because we can do something does not mean that we should. As a doctor, it is important to share the option of doing nothing as a legitimate treatment. In Mrs Deane's case, her main concern is hip pain, and shared decision-making with her consultant leads to a personalised approach which fulfils her specific needs.

The authors of this book have created a compendium of real-world cases that will challenge your medical acumen but will also challenge you to consider how you make decisions and the implications of those decisions for the lives of the people you are trying to help. Put yourself in the shoes of the fictional characters portrayed here – would you make the same choices as them? Each person that you interact with in your career will have their own values, needs and backstory. Your job is to encourage them to share these and listen to them when they do.

Dr Claire Macaulay, MD MRCP MBChB (Hons) BSc (Hons)
National Education Lead for Realistic Medicine
NHS Education for Scotland

Preface

Clinical medicine involves the intertwining of the lives of our patients with the health conditions that affect them. The course of an illness may change in a matter of seconds or hours, but many conditions progress and impact on the life of the patient for several months or even years.

With an increasing reliance on shift work, handovers and specialist referrals, seeing patients longitudinally throughout their illness is less common than it used to be. This has had a significant effect on our education and understanding of disease progression.

In the past, clinical case books have all too often provided a snapshot in time, looking at what happens to patients during a single episode. A short vignette leads directly to questions focused on identifying the diagnosis and the immediate treatment required. However, we feel that this ignores the way in which the process of disease affects both our patients and our care for them.

We feel the need for a new paradigm that looks at a longer time period, acknowledging the existence of developing clinical presentations and complications which may present over the course of several chronological episodes.

Therefore, we have developed a new style of clinical cases, presenting the cases with a timepoint structure, taking you step-by-step through key moments where new information becomes available, where investigations require action, or other moments where there is an important learning point.

We have created a series of clinical cases which cover a range of important medical conditions, constituting around five cases for each of the major internal medical specialities: cardiology, respiratory, gastroenterology, endocrinology, rheumatology and neurology. Other important areas such as oncology, infectious disease, toxicology, haematology, renal medicine and geriatrics are also covered to make up a total of 40 cases.

This book is designed to complement the learning of senior medical students and doctors early in their training. The scope includes scenarios based within hospital medicine but, importantly, also includes timepoints based in primary care and other community settings, as these are also places where junior doctors are expected to practice semi-autonomously.

We are deeply grateful for the help and support provided by a wide range of people in the development of this book. First and foremost, we would like to thank Dr Priti Dutta, a remarkable radiologist, who has contributed all of the outstanding radiology images included in this book. We thank those who have contributed partial clinical cases: Dr Tara Belcher, Dr Sophie Anne Elands, Dr Martin Glasser and Dr Rachel Tresman. We are also grateful to a number of people who have reviewed and edited content, including Dr Rebecca Bamford, Dr Katya Christodoulou, Dr Asma Fikree, Dr David Fisher, Louise Greenberg, Dr Catriona Hayes, Dr Rammya Mathew and Dr Yael Santhouse. Finally, we would like to thank our exceptional publishing team at CRC Press, Jo Koster and Julia Molloy, without whom this book would not have been possible.

Please inform us of any errors or anything else that you feel is worthy of comment for future editions.

Enjoy!

From the co-author team,
Andrew Solomon, Julia Anstey and Liora Wittner

Case 1

TIMEPOINT ⏱ 1

Mr Marsh, a 35-year-old teacher, has presented to the emergency department with a 2-day history of feeling weak in his legs and increasing difficulty walking. He is normally very active and plays football in his spare time; however, he is now finding it difficult to stand for more than a few minutes. Over the last day, he has started to suffer from pins and needles in his arms and feet and has pain in the rear of his neck. His bowels are functioning normally, but he has found that he is urinating more frequently than usual.

Prior to this, Mr Marsh has been generally well, apart from having 'food poisoning' 3 weeks ago. He has no significant past medical history, is currently on no medications and has no drug allergies. He does not smoke and drinks alcohol socially twice a week.

His observations are:

Respiratory rate: 14/min
Oxygen saturations: 99% on room air
Temperature: 36.8°C
Blood pressure: 112/74 mmHg
Heart rate: 72 bpm

On examination, Mr Marsh looks generally well. Cardiorespiratory and abdominal examinations are normal. A neurological examination of the upper limbs revealed asymmetric and variable power in the biceps, triceps and other muscle groups with altered sensation in an indistinct distribution across both arms. Examination of the lower limbs revealed increased tone, generalised reduced power (MRC 4+) amongst all muscle groups, normal to brisk reflexes, positive Babinski sign and generally impaired coordination. Rectal exam showed normal tone.

What investigations should be arranged?

- Urinalysis
- Bladder scan
- Bloods – FBC, U&Es, ESR, CRP, serum B12 and folate
- Lumbar puncture (preceded by CT head)
- MRI spinal cord
- MRI brain

Urinalysis was normal. A bladder scan showed an empty bladder.

Initial blood tests showed the following:

Venous blood results

Haemoglobin	140 g/L
White cell count	6.0×10^9/L
Platelets	253×10^9/L
Sodium	139 mmol/L
Potassium	4.4 mmol/L
Urea	6.1 mmol/L
Creatinine	90 µmol/L

A lumbar puncture was performed, which showed the following:

Lumbar puncture results

CSF fluid	Clear
CSF protein	1.2 g/L
CSF glucose	4.1 mmol/L
CSF cell count	High
Plasma glucose	4.8 mmol/L
Gram stain	No organisms

The MRI spine is shown in Figure 1.1.

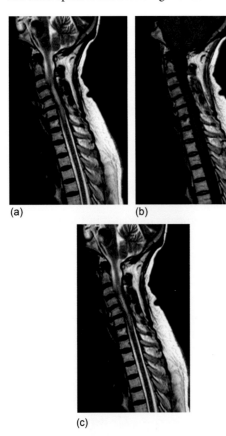

(a)   (b)

(c)

Figure 1.1 (a) Sagittal T2 MRI image through the cervical spine; (b) Sagittal T1 images through the cervical spine; (c) The red line demarcates a long segment of abnormal T2 increased signal within the cord. Imaging diagnostic criteria for transverse myelitis involve the demonstration of long segments (3 to 4 vertebral body heights or more) of spinal cord signal change, occupying more than two-thirds of the cross-sectional area of the cord. These may demonstrate variable patterns of enhancement and restricted diffusion

The MRI is reported as follows: *altered T2 and gadolinium enhanced signal within the spinal cord from the level of C3 to C7, with no suggestion of any compressive/space-occupying lesion.*

The clinical findings suggest a diagnosis of idiopathic transverse myelitis.

What are the diagnostic criteria for transverse myelitis?

The Transverse Myelitis Consortium Working Group suggests the following diagnostic criteria:

- Development of sensory, motor or autonomic dysfunction attributable to the spinal cord
- Bilateral signs and/or symptoms (though not necessarily symmetric)
- Clearly defined sensory level
- Exclusion of extra-axial compressive aetiology by neuroimaging (MRI or CT myelography)
- Inflammation of the spinal cord demonstrated by CSF pleocytosis, elevated IgG index or MRI gadolinium enhancement
- Progression to nadir between 4 hours and 21 days following the onset of symptoms

A significant percentage of patients presenting with a clinical pattern resembling transverse myelitis do not meet the inflammatory features of the criteria. It is important to note that the absence of inflammatory markers does not exclude transverse myelitis as the diagnosis.

How should Mr Marsh be managed?

First line: high-dose IV glucocorticoids for 3–5 days (either methylprednisolone, 1000 mg daily, or dexamethasone), alongside supportive care and acute rehabilitation.

Second line: plasmapheresis with supportive care and acute rehabilitation – for CNS demyelinating diseases that fail to respond to glucocorticoids.

TIMEPOINT 🕐 2

Four days after admission, Mr Marsh is seen on the morning ward round. He says he is starting to feel better already, and has been working with the physiotherapists to try to get his strength back. He has been having regular bedside capillary blood glucose monitoring after starting on steroids. The nurse notes that he had one value of 9.8 mmol/L yesterday evening, but all of the values preceding this had been <7.8 mmol/L.

The medical team tested his HbA1c which came back as 44 mmol/mol.

What does this HbA1c value mean?

- Mr Marsh is pre-diabetic. Diabetes can be diagnosed if HbA1c ≥48 mmol/mol. Pre-diabetes is diagnosed if the value is 42–47 mmol/mol
- Continue to monitor his capillary blood glucose
- Blood glucose may return to normal once he has finished his course of steroids

TIMEPOINT ⏱ 3

Three months later, Mr Marsh is back at work, but only standing in the classroom for brief periods and, in addition to ongoing regular physiotherapy, is doing gentle floor Pilates twice a week. His GP plans to arrange another HbA1c test. Mr Marsh, who has a relative with diabetes, thought that HbA1c values were usually expressed as a percentage. The GP explains that the standard is now to use the mmol/mol unit. The repeat HbA1c result is 42 mmol/mol (6%), which is reassuring.

What is the quick, simple method to convert HbA1c mmol/mol values to percentages?

It is the 'Minus 2 rule' – the exact digit percentages convert to mmol/mol, by subtracting 2 for the larger and smaller figure; for example; 9% = 75; 8% = 64; 7% = 53; 6% = 42.

TIMEPOINT ⏱ 4

A year later, Mr Marsh is referred to a neurology outpatient clinic, as he has noticed that he gets a tingling sensation down his back and legs when he looks down and is worried that this might be related to his previous symptoms.

What is the name of this phenomenon, and what might it indicate?

- Lhermitte's phenomenon – a tingling or 'electrical sensation' running down the back and into the limbs, elicited by neck flexion
- It is an indicator of demyelination
- This may suggest that he is developing multiple sclerosis; however, it can also be seen in a number of other neurological disorders including transverse myelitis, vitamin B12 deficiency (subacute combined degeneration of spinal cord) and compression of the cervical spinal cord among others

What are the long-term implications of transverse myelitis?

Recovery is likely to begin within 1–3 months; however, recovery is often only partial with 30–40% of patients retaining some degree of disability. Recurrence is also seen in 25–33% of patients with idiopathic transverse myelitis, while in disease-related transverse myelitis (connected to a wider neurological disease or other inflammatory conditions) this figure can rise to 70%.

There are some features that have been recognised to increase the chance of recurrence, which are often markers of a wider or more severe illness:

- Multiple lesions in the spinal cord on MRI
- Finding of brain lesions on MRI
- Autoantibody positivity for autoantibodies ANA, dsDNA, anti-phospholipid, c-ANCA
- Oligoclonal band positivity in the cerebrospinal fluid
- Positive test for NMO-IgG (anti-aquaporin-4) antibody

Those with severe acute complete transverse myelitis have the overall best prognosis as they are less likely to present with oligoclonal bands, less likely to suffer a relapse and have a low rate of transition to multiple sclerosis.

What is the risk of multiple sclerosis in such patients?

There is a notable risk of developing MS following an episode of transverse myelitis. This rate is between 5–30% over 3–5 years in patients in whom the initial cause is unknown, depending on whether it is acute complete (5–10%) or acute partial (10–30%). If at initial presentation of partial transverse myelitis there are already cranial lesions typical of MS seen on MRI, this rate goes up to 60–90% over 3–5 years.

What are the differential diagnoses of idiopathic transverse myelitis?

See Figure 1.2.

FURTHER READING

1. Proposed diagnostic criteria and nosology of acute transverse myelitis. Transverse Myelitis Consortium Working Group. *Neurology* 2002.27;59 (4):499–505.

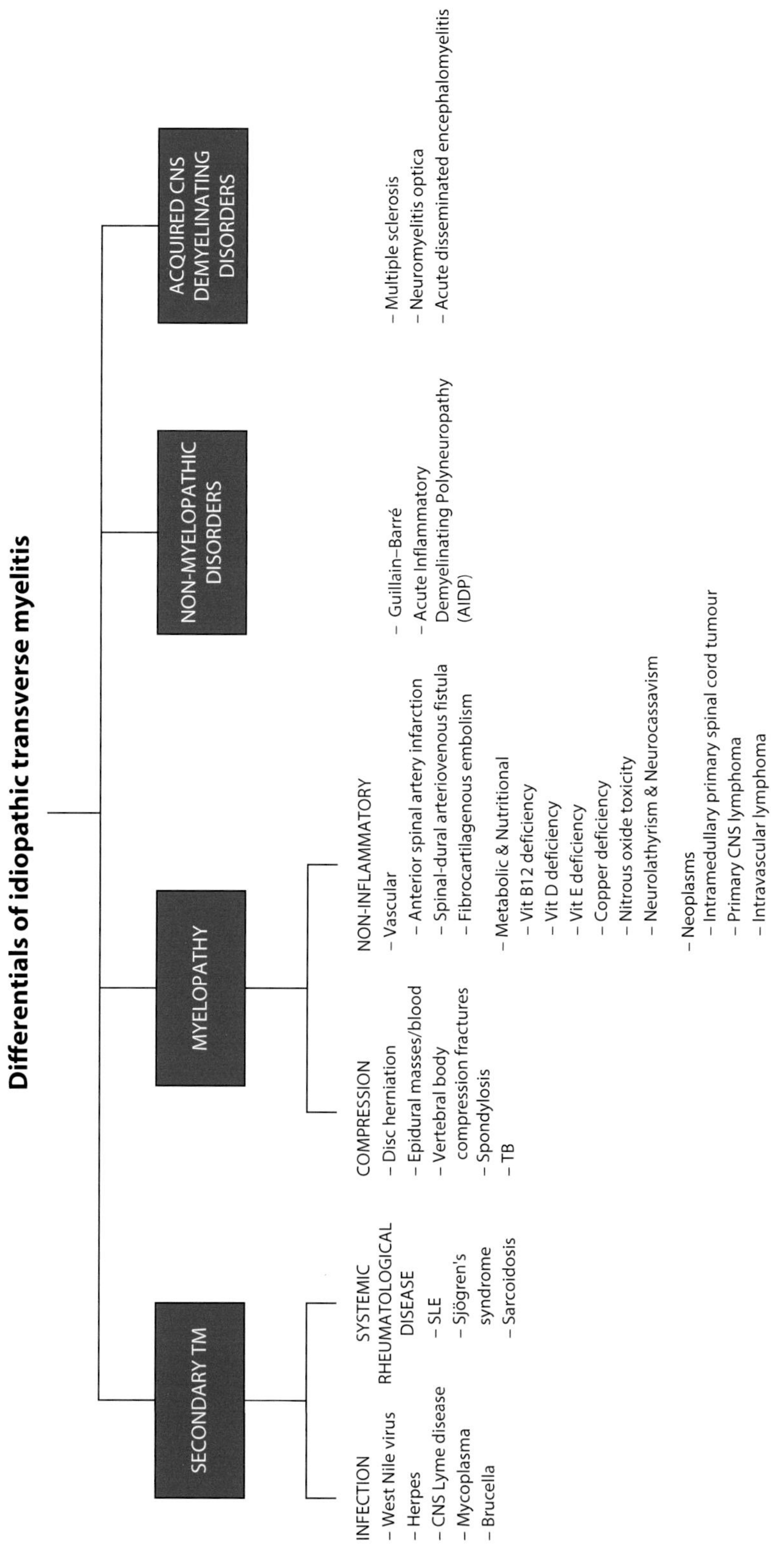

Differentials of idiopathic transverse myelitis

| | SECONDARY TM | MYELOPATHY | NON-MYELOPATHIC DISORDERS | ACQUIRED CNS DEMYELINATING DISORDERS |

SECONDARY TM

INFECTION
- West Nile virus
- Herpes
- CNS Lyme disease
- Mycoplasma
- Brucella

SYSTEMIC RHEUMATOLOGICAL DISEASE
- SLE
- Sjögren's syndrome
- Sarcoidosis

MYELOPATHY

COMPRESSION
- Disc herniation
- Epidural masses/blood
- Vertebral body compression fractures
- Spondylosis
- TB

NON-INFLAMMATORY
- Vascular
  - Anterior spinal artery infarction
  - Spinal-dural arteriovenous fistula
  - Fibrocartilagenous embolism
- Metabolic & Nutritional
  - Vit B12 deficiency
  - Vit D deficiency
  - Vit E deficiency
  - Copper deficiency
  - Nitrous oxide toxicity
  - Neurolathyrism & Neurocassavism
- Neoplasms
  - Intramedullary primary spinal cord tumour
  - Primary CNS lymphoma
  - Intravascular lymphoma

NON-MYELOPATHIC DISORDERS

- Guillain–Barré
- Acute Inflammatory Demyelinating Polyneuropathy (AIDP)

ACQUIRED CNS DEMYELINATING DISORDERS

- Multiple sclerosis
- Neuromyelitis optica
- Acute disseminated encephalomyelitis

Figure 1.2 The differential diagnoses for idiopathic transverse myelitis.

Case 2

Mr Patel, a 60-year-old businessman, collapsed at home and was brought into the emergency department by ambulance. At 11 am this morning he had been working from home, when his wife heard a thud and rushed into the room to find that he had collapsed and was unconscious. He describes feeling light-headed for a few seconds before 'blacking out'. His wife thinks he was unconscious for about 30 seconds before waking up. He did not bite his tongue or make jerky movements and was not incontinent of urine or feces. Upon waking, he was particularly short of breath and his lips looked blue. He has had a cough for the past week.

His past medical history includes obesity, hypertension and high cholesterol, for which he takes atorvastatin, amlodipine and ramipril. He had a previous deep-vein thrombosis 4 years ago. He has recently been under a lot of extra family and professional stress, making several long journeys to business meetings in the last few weeks. He has no allergies, drinks occasionally and smokes 8 cigarettes per day. He went to see his practice nurse for a health check 6 weeks ago, where they discussed weight loss and smoking cessation. He has had no recent trauma or surgery.

On examination, Mr Patel's observations are:

Respiratory rate: 26/min
Oxygen saturations: 92% on high-flow oxygen
   (79% before oxygen administered)
Temperature: 36.8°C
Blood pressure: 85/65 mmHg
Heart rate: 110 bpm

Cardiorespiratory examination reveals a raised JVP and loud S2 heart sound. His fingertips and lips have a blue discolouration. Lung fields are clear on auscultation, percussion and vocal fremitus are normal and equal. He has cool peripheries. There are no other examination findings of note.

What investigations might be ordered and why?

- ECG – to look for a cardiac cause for collapse or evidence of pulmonary embolism (PE)
- Routine blood tests including D-dimer and troponin – to look for MI or PE
- ABG – may show reduced PaO_2 and/or $PaCO_2$
- Chest X-ray – to look for lung pathology, e.g. tension pneumothorax, or may show Westermark's Triad
- Echocardiography – for structural abnormalities, e.g. aortic stenosis
- CTPA – to investigate for PE

Investigations

Initial blood tests showed the following:

Venous and arterial blood results

D-Dimer	3867 ng/mL
pH	7.44
$PaCO_2$	4.8 kPa
PaO_2	7.7 kPa
HCO_3	22 mmol/L
Base excess	2 mmol/L

The ECG shows a dominant R wave in V1 and sinus tachycardia.

DOI: 10.1201/9781351257725-2

What would initial management involve?

- A DRABCDE approach. Assess haemodynamic stability and focus on stabilising the patient while carrying out diagnostic tests

Given that Mr Patel is haemodynamically unstable (systolic BP <90 mmHg for >15 mins), what would be your next steps in management?

- Administer oxygen (target saturations ≥90%)/mechanical ventilation if necessary
- IV fluid resuscitation
- Consider IV vasopressor therapy – where adequate perfusion is not restored with IV fluid resuscitation. Noradrenaline is the preferred drug, as it is less likely to cause tachycardia (exacerbating hypotension) than dopamine and adrenaline
- Anticoagulation – following suitable risk stratification
- Arrange CTPA

If clinical suspicion for PE is high – taking into account bleeding risk and expected timing of diagnostic tests – immediate anticoagulation is advised along with prompt imaging (CTPA where available) to confirm. Careful clinical judgement must be used as the optimal agent will depend on the haemodynamic stability of the patient, presence of risk factors and comorbidities and anticipated need for later procedures or thrombolysis. If the patient is too unstable for scanning, and a portable perfusion scan is not available, an echocardiogram is advised to aid a presumptive diagnosis of PE before administering systemic thrombolytic therapy.

If clinical suspicion for PE is only low or moderate, empiric thrombolysis is not justified before confirmation of diagnosis, and management should follow that of a haemodynamically stable patient.

Wells' Score

In patients that are haemodynamically stable, the Wells' Score for PE can be used to determine the clinical probability of a pulmonary embolus. An alternative prediction score is the Geneva score.

Clinical signs or symptoms of DVT	+3
PE is top diagnosis OR equally likely	+3
Heart rate >100	+1.5
Immobilisation at least 3 days OR surgery in previous 4 weeks	+1.5
Previous, objectively diagnosed PE or DVT	+1.5
Haemoptysis	+1
Malignancy with treatment within 6 months or palliative	+1

- 0–4 points – PE unlikely (12.1% incidence of PE). Consider D-dimer
  - If D-dimer negative consider stopping work-up
  - If D-dimer positive, consider CTPA
- >4 points – PE likely (37.1% incidence of PE). Consider CTPA

Even in patients with a low risk of PE, if bleeding risk is low, anticoagulant therapy is indicated as follows:

Initial anticoagulation (0–10 days)

- Given as soon as possible according to local guidelines – gold standard is within one hour of clinical suspicion of PE unless contraindicated
- This can be stopped if PE is excluded as a diagnosis

Long-term anticoagulation (10 days–3 months)

- Long-term therapy given beyond the initial phase once PE confirmed
- Usually involves changing agents from parenteral to oral administration for long-term use

- Continue for 3 months for provoked VTE
- Continue for 6–12 months for persisting risk factors or unprovoked VTE

Indefinite anticoagulation

- Some patients will need to be on anticoagulation indefinitely depending on several factors, e.g. provoked vs. unprovoked event, risk of bleeding or recurrence, presence of risk factors (e.g. transient or persistent), patient preference

Mr Patel has a CTPA which shows he has a massive pulmonary embolus. See Figure 2.1.

Mr Patel is still unstable and has a low risk of bleeding, therefore thrombolysis should be administered. Thrombolysis should only be used for haemodynamically unstable patients. If thrombolysis were to be contraindicated, an embolectomy can be considered if appropriate expertise is accessible. Although it is commonplace for intravenous thrombolysis to be available, catheter-directed thrombolysis is now being offered in certain centres.

TIMEPOINT ⏱ 2

One hour after the CTPA scan, Mr Patel is given thrombolysis and has very careful monitoring of observations, before, during and after the treatment.

Approximately 2 hours post-thrombolysis, Mr Patel's cardiovascular stability has shown a marked improvement as demonstrated by the observations below:

Respiratory rate: 20/min
Oxygen saturations: 96% on 2 litres oxygen
Temperature: 36.7°C
Blood pressure: 112/74 mmHg
Heart rate: 85 bpm

What is the likely risk of recurrence of a PE?

Risk of recurrence is greatest within the first 2 weeks after the primary event, but lies at around 2% with adequate anticoagulant therapy. For this reason, it is important to rapidly achieve therapeutic anticoagulation levels.

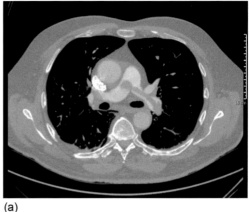

(a)

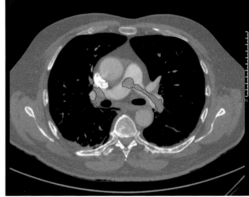

(b)

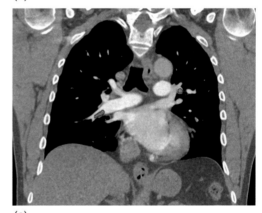

(c)

Figure 2.1 Contrast enhanced computed tomography (CT) images in the axial (a and b) and coronal planes (c). There is a saddle embolus, which extends into lobar pulmonary arteries, outlined in red (b and c).

What is the next step in Mr Patel's management?

Start warfarin, or a DOAC and give him heparin until his INR/steady state of DOAC reaches a therapeutic level.

TIMEPOINT ⏰ 3

The next morning, Mr Patel is seen on the post-take ward round. He is now feeling much better and is sitting up in bed. His pulse is now 86 bpm and blood pressure 130/80 mmHg.

What are the long-term implications of having a PE?

Following this episode, Mr Patel will require regular follow-up to monitor the following:

- Monitor therapeutic levels of INR (target 2–3) if on warfarin, although large numbers of patients will now be offered a DOAC such as rivaroxaban or apixaban
- He has been given advice to lose weight – this can affect the half-life of the anticoagulant used, and should therefore be monitored
- Early recurrence particularly within the first 2 weeks following diagnosis

- Late complications including chronic thromboembolic pulmonary hypertension (CTEPH), as well as new symptoms of recurrence of PE or DVT
- Adverse effects of medications
- Bleeding risk
- The need to be vigilant for, and possibly consider suitable screening towards underlying predisposing risk factors

TIMEPOINT ⏰ 4

After 6 months, Mr Patel is seen in the anticoagulation clinic. He is still taking his warfarin, but he has been getting a skin rash that he thinks is associated with it and is struggling to attend all the monitoring appointments due to his busy work schedule. He is wondering if there is an alternative medication that he could take. There are alternative drugs from the DOAC family that tend to have fewer side effects and need monitoring less frequently, e.g. rivaroxaban or apixaban.

What are the commonly used anticoagulant therapies available?

See Table 2.1.

Table 2.1 A summary of the anticoagulants that can be used

Anticoagulants					
Parenteral			Oral		
Indirect	Direct		Indirect	Direct	
Unfractionated heparin (UFH)	Thrombin inhibitors	Factor Xa inhibitors	Warfarin	Thrombin inhibitors	Factor Xa inhibitors
LMWH Fondaparinux M118	Hirudin Bivalirudin Argatroban	Otamixaban		Dabigatran	Rivaroxaban Apixaban Edoxaban
LMW heparin • Preferred in DVT in pregnancy and active malignancy. Fondaparinux • Monitoring not required. • Contraindicated in severe renal dysfunction.	Rarely used in clinical practice.	Rarely used in clinical practice.	• Preferred for patients with renal insufficiency. • But needs regular INR monitoring and higher bleeding risk. • Antidotes for warfarin-related bleeding more readily available.	• Preferred for haemodynamically stable, non-pregnant, no severe renal insufficiency or active cancer. • Reduced need for monitoring. • Similar efficacy to warfarin. • Lower risk of bleeding. • HOWEVER, experience with antidotes is limited. • NOT SUITABLE for patients with haemodynamically unstable PE.	

Case 3

TIMEPOINT 1

Mr Riley, a 60-year-old gentleman, is brought to the emergency department after being found looking unsteady. His brother is visiting, having not seen him for 6 months, and says that he looks dishevelled and has lost a lot of weight, and he is particularly worried about him given recent events. Mr Riley was made redundant a year ago and has been living alone for several months following a divorce. He does not declare any significant past medical history, denies drinking excessively and says that he has certainly never taken illicit drugs. He has no allergies, no regular medication and does not smoke.

His observations are:

Respiratory rate: 14/min
Oxygen saturations: 99% on room air
Temperature: 36.5°C
Blood pressure: 118/75 mmHg
Heart rate: 82 bpm

On examination, Mr Riley is alert but looks unkempt. His speech is slurred at times and contains repetitive content. On neurological examination, he has an intention tremor and dysdiadokokinesia. On examination of vision, he has difficulty focussing on specific items and appears to have disconjugate eye movements on upgaze.

What investigations would be indicated?

- Bloods – FBC, U&Es, LFTs, haematinics, red cell transketolase
- CT head
- MRI head

Mr Riley's blood tests come back showing:

MCV 104 fL
Red cell transketolase – low

What does a low red cell transketolase indicate?

- Low red cell transketolase indicates a thiamine (vitamin B1) deficiency
- Transketolase is an enzyme in the pentose–phosphate pathway, with thiamine and magnesium as its cofactors. Thiamine is vital to cellular energy production, and therefore any deficiency tends to affect the most active tissues first – brain, nervous system and heart

TIMEPOINT 2

Around 2 hours after arrival, Mr Riley becomes tachycardic, sweaty and seems particularly agitated, making multiple attempts to get off of the trolley.

What might be the cause of this?

- Alcohol withdrawal

What is an appropriate management plan?

- Provide parenteral administration of thiamine and chlordiazepoxide as appropriate
- Left untreated, Wernicke encephalopathy can lead to coma and death and therefore diagnostic testing should not delay treatment. Prompt administration of treatment should result in an improvement in ocular signs within hours to days, with confusion subsiding over days to weeks (Figure 3.1)

DOI: 10.1201/9781351257725-3

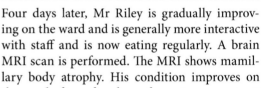

> **ENCEPHALOPATHY**
> - Profound disorientation
> - Indifference
> - Inattentiveness
> - Impaired memory and learning
> - Agitated delirium due to associated alcohol withdrawal
> - If left untreated, lethargy, coma & death

> **OCULOMOTOR**
> - Nystagmus – oculomotor lesion (most common finding)
> - Lateral rectus palsy – abducens lesion (almost always bilateral)
> - Conjugate gaze palsies – vestibular nuclei lesion
>
> These symptoms usually occur in combination rather than alone. Sluggish or unequal pupils may be present.

> **GAIT ATAXIA**
> May exhibit a wide-based gait with slow short-spaced steps. Likely a combination of the following:
> - Polyneuropathy
> - Cerebellar – pathology restricted to anterior and superior vermis, making ataxia of the legs or arms uncommon, in contrast to alcoholic cerebellar degeneration when it is very common
> - Vestibular dysfunction

Figure 3.1 The classic triad of Wernicke encephalopathy.

Administering dextrose in thiamine deficiency

The administration of dextrose in thiamine deficiency can be very harmful. Glucose oxidation is a thiamine-intensive process that may drive insufficient circulating vitamin B1 and therefore lead to neurologic injury. Thiamine should always be administered before glucose.

What are the potential complications of Wernicke encephalopathy?

- Hypotension
- Hypothermia
- Alcohol withdrawal
- Acute precipitation of WE
- Congestive heart failure
- Gastrointestinal beriberi
- Lactic acidosis
- Worsening with administration of dextrose in thiamine deficiency

TIMEPOINT 🕐 3

Four days later, Mr Riley is gradually improving on the ward and is generally more interactive with staff and is now eating regularly. A brain MRI scan is performed. The MRI shows mamillary body atrophy. His condition improves on the ward after a few days of ongoing assessment by physiotherapy and occupational therapy colleagues leading to a successful discharge.

What is the significance of mamillary body atrophy?

Mamillary body atrophy occurs in thiamine deficiency and in the conditions associated with Wernicke's and Korsakoff syndrome. It can also be seen in other forms of liver failure, schizophrenia and some other neurodegenerative conditions.

TIMEPOINT 🕐 4

Six months later, Mr Riley was trying to carry cups and saucers at a family event, when he was noted to have a tremor. His GP referred him to the neurology clinic. The neurologist felt that the tremor could be described as benign essential tremor but, on further cognitive assessment, detected a degree of memory impairment.

What chronic neurological condition can occur as a consequence of Wernicke encephalopathy?

* Korsakoff syndrome

Korsakoff syndrome

Korsakoff syndrome is characterised by marked deficits in anterograde and retrograde amnesia and apathy, with relative preservation of long-term memory and other cognitive skills. It is a late neuropsychiatric manifestation of Wernicke encephalopathy and is seen most frequently in alcohol abusers after an episode of WE. Patients rarely recover from Korsakoff syndrome and usually need social support or a chronic care facility.

Mr Riley will require long-term follow-up coordinated by his GP, including:

* Referral for advice from a dietician

* Referral to local alcohol liaison team/other alcohol services/charities
* Interval liver function tests – always bear in mind that normal LFTs do not exclude cirrhosis. Refer for liver ultrasound if appropriate

There are a number of charities that can help with alcohol dependency and addiction.

Alcoholics Anonymous (AA) is one of the most well-known charities, which holds meetings all around the country, every week, to provide moral support to those with alcohol problems through their 12-step programme. The following are all helpful Web pages for advice and support on how to cut down on alcohol consumption:

* www.nhs.uk/Livewell/alcohol/Pages/Alcohol support.aspx
* www.al-anonuk.org.uk
* www.addaction.org.uk
* www.adfam.org.uk
* www.nacoa.org.uk
* www.smartrecovery.org.uk

Alcohol use can be associated with other psychosocial issues, including drug use, social and housing issues, and mental health conditions. It is important to consider community referrals to other local services and charities that may be of benefit.

Case 4

TIMEPOINT 1

Mrs Morley, a 77-year-old retired secretary, presents to the GP after feeling tired and generally unwell for the past 4 weeks. She feels hot and feverish, particularly at night, and feels that her clothes are looser than they used to be. She does not have a cough or shortness of breath and only complains of pain in her right knee. She also had a minor procedure at the dentist last month.

Her past medical history includes high cholesterol and hypertension. She lives with her husband, and normally mobilises independently. She has no recent history of foreign travel, gave up smoking 23 years ago and only drinks alcohol occasionally. She takes no regular medication and has no drug allergies.

Her observations are:

Respiratory rate: 12/min
Oxygen saturations: 99% on room air
Temperature: 37.9°C
Blood pressure: 170/74 mmHg
Heart rate: 78 bpm

On examination, Mrs Morley is alert and awake. On cardiorespiratory examination, there is a harsh ejection systolic murmur, heard best at the left sternal edge, followed by an early diastolic murmur heard best in full expiration. All other examination findings are normal.

What investigations would be appropriate to perform?

- Urinalysis
- FBC, U&Es, CRP, LFTs, TFTs
- Tumour markers
- Blood cultures – three sets from different sites (preferably before commencing antibiotics)
- Chest X-ray
- ECG
- Echocardiogram

What are the criteria for the most likely diagnosis?

The diagnosis of infective endocarditis is definite when: (a) a microorganism is demonstrated by culture of a specimen from a vegetation, an embolism or an intracardiac abscess; (b) active endocarditis is confirmed by histological examination of the vegetation or intracardiac abscess; (c) two major clinical criteria, one major and three minor criteria, or five minor criteria are met (Table 4.1).

What is the most likely organism the blood cultures will grow?

- *Streptococcus viridans*

(Note: *Staphylococcus aureus* is now the most common cause of infective endocarditis, but given the recent dental history in this case, *Streptococcus viridans* remains the most likely.)

TIMEPOINT 2

The next day, Mrs Morley has both transthoracic and transoesophageal echocardiograms, alongside ward round review and further microbiology advice regarding appropriate antibiotic treatment.

DOI: 10.1201/9781351257725-4

Table 4.1 The modified Duke Criteria for infective endocarditis

Major criteria	Minor criteria
Positive blood culture for infective endocarditis: as defined by the recovery of a typical microorganism from two separate blood cultures in the absence of a primary focus (Viridans streptococci, *Abiotrophia* species and *Granulicatella* species; *Streptococcus bovis*, HACEK group or community-acquired *Staphylococcus aureus* or *Enterococcus* species)	**Predisposition**: predisposing heart condition or IV drug use
Persistently positive blood cultures: defined as the recovery of a microorganism consistent with endocarditis from either blood samples obtained more than 12 hours apart or all three or a majority of four or more separate blood samples, with the first and last obtained at least 1 hour apart	**Fever**: temperature >38°C (100.4°F)
A positive serological test for Q fever: with an immunofluorescence assay showing phase 1 IgG antibodies at a titre >1:800	**Vascular phenomena**: major arterial emboli, septic pulmonary infarcts, mycotic aneurysm, intracranial haemorrhage, conjunctival haemorrhages, Janeway's lesion
Echocardiographic evidence of endocardial involvement: • An oscillating intracardiac mass on the valve or supporting structures, in the path of regurgitant jets, or on implanted material in the absence of an alternative anatomical explanation • An abscess • New partial dehiscence of prosthetic valve	**Immunologic phenomena**: glomerulonephritis, Osler's nodes, Roth's spots, rheumatoid factor
New valvular regurgitation	**Microbiological evidence**: a positive blood culture but not meeting a major criterion,* or serological evidence of an active infection with an organism that can cause infective endocarditis
	Echocardiogram: findings consistent with infective endocarditis but not meeting a major criterion

Excludes single positive cultures for coagulase-negative staphylococci, diphtheroids and organisms that do not commonly cause endocarditis.

Which valve would be expected to show a significant abnormality?

• Aortic valve

Transoesophageal ultrasound showed a large vegetation on the aortic valve.

This would be consistent with infective endocarditis.

How could Mrs Morley be managed?

• Treatment for acute native valve confirmed endocarditis with penicillin-susceptible viridans group streptococci
  • 4–6-week course of antibiotics: beta-lactam plus gentamicin, or vancomycin alone (see local hospital guidelines)
  • Weekly ECG monitoring to monitor PR interval

How it's done: Transoesophageal echocardiogram

A specialised ultrasound probe is passed down the patient's oesophagus, allowing very clear images of heart structures and valves (particularly those posteriorly) to be taken.

It allows more detailed pictures to be taken than a normal echocardiogram.

The throat is first sprayed with local anaesthetic to numb it and suppress the gag reflex. A mild sedative is administered through an IV line in the patient's arm. An ECG is attached to the patient's chest. The doctor passes the thin probe through the patient's mouth and down their throat, and they are asked to swallow it as it goes down. The probe sends out ultrasound waves, creating a picture that can be seen on a screen. This will take 10–15 minutes. Once the doctor is finished, the probe and ECG leads are removed. The patient is monitored until fully awake, but can then usually get up and leave the hospital.

Patients may experience some difficulty swallowing for a few hours after the test, and may have a sore throat for a couple of days. Due to the sedative given it is also important for the patient not to drink for a couple of hours.

- CT imaging of aortic root if any suggestion of abscess formation
- +/– Surgery

Mrs Morley is started on amoxicillin and low-dose gentamicin, but after *Streptococcus viridans* is confirmed on blood cultures, she is switched on to benzylpenicillin for 4 weeks.

TIMEPOINT ⏱ 3

Two days later, Mrs Morley develops a widespread maculopapular rash and is particularly itchy. The doctor seeing her on the ward round is concerned that this may be a drug reaction.

How would this clinical scenario be managed?

- Assume this is a drug reaction and stop benzylpenicillin. Seek microbiology advice for a suitable alternative
- Record the penicillin allergy status in the medical record/primary care notes
- Administer supportive therapy – oral antihistamines, topical steroids and moisturising lotions
- Monitor the progression of the rash and for any other symptoms

TIMEPOINT ⏱ 4

Four weeks later, the echocardiogram is repeated in the final week of antibiotic therapy and shows the aortic valve has deteriorated with severe aortic regurgitation. The cardiology team meets with Mrs Morley and through a process of shared decision-making, it is decided that an aortic valve replacement would be suitable. They arrange an MDT discussion with the cardiothoracic surgeons regarding an open procedure vs. a transcatheter aortic valve implantation (TAVI). Given Mrs Morley's good functional status and advice from the MDT discussion, she opts to have an open aortic valve replacement.

What are the potential complications of infective endocarditis?

See Figure 4.1.

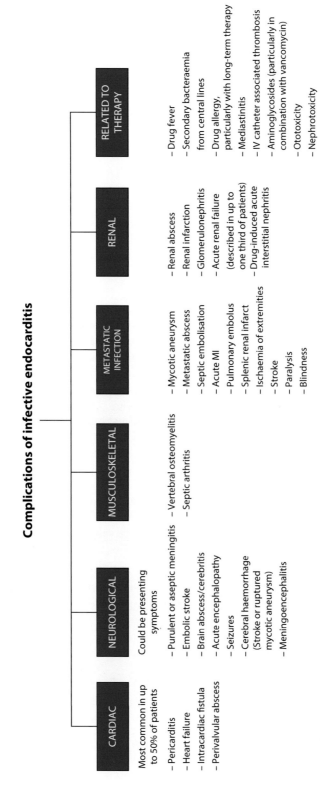

Complications of infective endocarditis

CARDIAC

Most common in up to 50% of patients

- Pericarditis
- Heart failure
- Intracardiac fistula
- Perivalvular abscess

NEUROLOGICAL

Could be presenting symptoms

- Purulent or aseptic meningitis
- Embolic stroke
- Brain abscess/cerebritis
- Acute encephalopathy
- Seizures
- Cerebral haemorrhage (Stroke or ruptured mycotic aneurysm)
- Meningoencephalitis

MUSCULOSKELETAL

- Vertebral osteomyelitis
- Septic arthritis

METASTATIC INFECTION

- Mycotic aneurysm
- Metastatic abscess
- Septic embolisation
- Acute MI
- Pulmonary embolus
- Splenic renal infarct
- Ischaemia of extremities
- Stroke
- Paralysis
- Blindness

RENAL

- Renal abscess
- Renal infarction
- Glomerulonephritis
- Acute renal failure (described in up to one third of patients)
- Drug-induced acute interstitial nephritis

RELATED TO THERAPY

- Drug fever
- Secondary bacteraemia from central lines
- Drug allergy, particularly with long-term therapy
- Mediastinitis
- IV catheter associated thrombosis
- Aminoglycosides (particularly in combination with vancomycin)
- Ototoxicity
- Nephrotoxicity

Figure 4.1 Complications of infective endocarditis.

Case 5

TIMEPOINT ⏱ 1

Mr Larsson, a 26-year-old stockbroker, has presented to the GP with a sore neck. He first noticed it was painful while shaving, roughly 2 weeks ago; however, it has felt more tender in the last week. He usually weighs himself at the gym and has noticed that he has lost 2 kg in weight since the pain started. He also describes feeling increasingly agitated at times, but has been having a particularly stressful time at work. He has had a new line manager for the last 3 months and has been sleeping less well than usual. He gets palpitations most days, especially before board meetings.

On examination, Mr Larsson has a tender anterior neck, but no palpable masses or nodules.

His observations are:

Respiratory rate: 14/min
Oxygen saturations: 99% on room air
Temperature: 37.8°C
Blood pressure: 118/77 mmHg
Heart rate: 52 bpm

His GP sends him for some blood tests.

Which investigations would be appropriate to order?

- Blood tests – including FBC, U&Es, LFTs, ESR, TFTs

A few days later, the blood test results come back. The FBC, U&E and LFTs were all normal.

Venous blood results

TSH	<0.03 mU/L (0.4–4.5 mU/L)
ESR	92 mm/hr (<20 mm/hr)
Thyroid peroxidase antibody – TPOAb	40 IU/mL (0–60 IU/mL)
Thyroid-stimulating immunoglobulin – TSI	0.3 IU/L (<0.56 IU/L)

What do these results show?

The results suggest hyperthyroidism but with normal TPO and TSI antibody status, making the likely cause of the condition a form of inflammatory thyroiditis. It is less likely to be autoimmune, as in conditions such as Graves' disease, it is common for antibodies to be positive, particularly thyroid-stimulating immunoglobulin.

What are the differential diagnoses in patients with altered TSH and/ or T4?

The differential diagnosis in thyroid conditions depends on the history, examination and investigations, none of which should be clinically interpreted in isolation. However, it can be useful to list the probable range of diagnoses based on whether TSH or T4 is reduced, normal or elevated; see Table 5.1.

With regard to the most likely diagnosis, how might Mr Larsson be managed?

- Supportive management
- NSAIDs work well to control the pain; if these are not sufficient, pain management can be stepped up to opioids. High-dose

DOI: 10.1201/9781351257725-5

Table 5.1 Causes of thyroid function test abnormalities

	Raised TSH	Normal TSH	Low TSH
Raised T4	TSH-secreting pituitary tumour (TSHoma) Thyroid hormone resistance syndrome Acute psychosis Thyroxine replacement therapy Assay error	TSH-secreting pituitary tumour (TSHoma)	Graves' disease Toxic thyroid adenoma 'hot nodule' Toxic multinodular goitre Subacute or granulomatous thyroiditis Excess thyroid ingestion Iodine-induced hyperthyroidism Drugs, e.g. amiodarone, excess iodine
Normal T4	Subclinical hypothyroidism Recovery from non-thyroid illness Poor adherence with thyroxine replacement or its malabsorption Drugs promoting increased metabolism of thyroid hormone, e.g. amiodarone Assay error	Normal	Subclinical hyperthyroidism Sick euthyroid syndrome Drugs that inhibit pituitary TSH secretion Pregnancy – first trimester Drugs, e.g. steroids, dopamine
Low T4	Hashimoto's thyroiditis Thyroidectomy Irradiation	Secondary or central hypothyroidism Drugs that increase hepatic metabolism of T4 Assay error	Secondary or central hypothyroidism Sick euthyroid syndrome

corticosteroids can be used if pain is severe and unrelieved by NSAIDs plus opioids
- β-blockers can be used for symptomatic relief of tachycardia, anxiety or tremor

TIMEPOINT ⏰ 2

Three weeks later, Mr Larsson comes back to the GP practice. He is now concerned that he is feeling very tired and lethargic. The GP agrees to ensure repeat blood tests are arranged and then sets up an electronic Web-based consultation to seek advice based on the results from one of the local endocrinologists.

His thyroid function tests are repeated and show the following:

T4 13 pmol/L (12–22 pmol/L)
TSH 5.1 mU/L (0.4–4.5 mU/L)

How might this scenario be managed in consideration of the changing TFT result?

- Continue to monitor thyroid function tests – follow-up in 2 weeks' time to recheck thyroid function tests
- If Mr Larsson were to become particularly symptomatic, and/or if the test results show biochemical hypothyroidism consider starting him on a 6-month trial of levothyroxine

TIMEPOINT ⏱ 3

Six weeks later, a planned clinic follow-up takes place after another set of thyroid function tests. His blood tests show the following:

T4 11.7 pmol/L (12–22 pmol/L)
TSH 4.9 mU/L (0.4–4.5 mU/L)

The T4 value is minimally below and TSH slightly above the reference range. The decision is taken to repeat the blood tests in a further 2–4 weeks to determine the direction of the thyroid function status.

Should thyroxine treatment be initiated in people with normal T4 and raised TSH?

This situation is the focus of much discussion and is known as subclinical hypothyroidism. In some cases, thyroid function tests revert to values within the reference ranges on later testing, but in some this is not the case. It can be a stepping stone to genuine hypothyroidism. Factors thought to be potentially linked more closely to a hypothyroid picture are positive TPO antibody status and dyslipidaemia. In general, international guidelines do recommend the use of thyroxine if the TSH is above range in patients aiming to conceive or who are pregnant, aiming for a TSH in the low-normal range. In other patients, it is more common to reassess as to whether a sustained rise in TSH and lowering of T4 takes place.

TIMEPOINT ⏱ 4

Eight weeks later, Mr Larsson returns to endocrine clinic with the opportunity to discuss the most recent blood tests which show the following:

T4 9 pmol/L (12–22 pmol/L)
TSH 11 mU/L (0.4–4.5 mU/L)

These data continue the trend as determined by the preceding blood tests and show definitive hypothyroidism as seen with a clearly low T4 and raised TSH.

The endocrinologist decides to initiate thyroxine at a dose of 50 mcg once daily to be taken early in the morning. Information is provided to Mr Larsson about the need to take thyroxine long term and the ongoing requirement for blood test monitoring.

What is De Quervain's thyroiditis?

This is a form of inflammatory thyroid condition – often commencing with self-limiting transient hyperthyroidism, usually viral in origin.

Apart from toxicosis, there is usually fever, malaise and pain in the neck with tachycardia and local thyroid tenderness. This sequence of clinical findings is consistent with de Quervain's thyroiditis.

Symptoms are often mild and short-lived. Normalisation of function usually occurs within 2–8 weeks. However, patients with symptomatic hypothyroidism may require treatment with levothyroxine.

Treatment of the acute phase is usually with aspirin or other NSAIDs, with short-term prednisolone in severely symptomatic cases.

FURTHER READING

1. NICE Guideline; www.nice.org.uk/guidance/ng145; Published November 2019.

Case 6

TIMEPOINT 1

Mrs Leigh is a 60-year-old Caucasian architect who has recently seen the practice nurse at her local GP surgery for a routine blood pressure check.

She has a history of gout but is otherwise well. She has no family history of cardiovascular disease. Her BMI is 32, and she is a non-smoker. She occasionally drinks alcohol at parties, but not on a regular basis. She lives with her husband and two adult children.

Her blood pressure was 168/108 mmHg and then 164/107 mmHg (two readings were taken) when checked by the practice nurse.

What should be done at this stage?

- Ambulatory blood pressure measurements (ABPM) or home blood pressure measurements (HBPM)
- QRISK2 cardiovascular assessment
- Check for target organ damage
  - Urine dip for haematuria
  - Albumin: creatinine ratio
  - Blood tests for HbA1c, electrolytes, creatinine, eGFR, total and HDL cholesterol
  - Fundoscopy for hypertensive retinopathy
  - 12 lead ECG

The practice nurse arranges the blood test, books Mrs Leigh for an ECG and urine testing and provides Mrs Leigh with a specific blood pressure machine to allow her to do ABPM.

ABPM, HBPM and 'white coat' hypertension

- ABPM should be offered to confirm the diagnosis if clinic blood pressure is between 140/90 mmHg and 180/120 mmHg
- The patients wear a blood pressure cuff continuously for 24 or 72 hours and readings are recorded automatically. There should be at least two readings per hour during the patient's normal waking hours
- At least 14 daytime readings should be used to calculate an average daytime ABPM
- Hypertension is confirmed if the daytime average ABPM is above 135/85 mmHg
- ABPM is useful to distinguish between genuine and 'white coat' hypertension (where there is a discrepancy of more than 20/10 mmHg between clinic measurements and average daytime ABPM), which helps to prevent over-diagnosis and the use of medication unnecessarily
- ABPM may be inaccurate if the patient has an arrhythmia
- ABPM cannot be used to detect postural hypotension unless the patient keeps a careful event diary
- If ABPM is unsuitable or unavailable, HBPM can be used, where the patient checks their own blood pressure at home (two readings, twice a day for 7 days)
- If hypertension is not diagnosed, blood pressure should be rechecked at least every 5 years

Later in the week, the GP reviews the results, which shows that Mrs Leigh's average daytime blood pressure on ABPM is 145/92 mmHg. He books Mrs Leigh into his clinic to discuss blood pressure control.

What dietary and lifestyle advice might Mrs Leigh be given?

- Encourage a balanced and healthy diet, in particular reducing salt intake
- Reduce caffeine and alcohol intake
- Encourage exercise
- Encourage smoking cessation and provide smoking cessation support if necessary

On the basis of the ABPM results, should Mrs Leigh be started on anti-hypertensive treatment?

- This is stage 1 hypertension in a patient under 80 years
  - (Clinic blood pressure: between 140/90 mmHg and 159/99 mmHg, and ABPM/HBPM: between 135/85 mmHg and 149/94 mmHg)
- Stage 1 hypertension should be treated if the patient also has one or more of the following
  - Target organ damage
  - Cardiovascular disease or an estimated 10-year risk of ≥10% (using QRISK2)
  - Renal disease
  - Diabetes
- Mrs Leigh does not have any of the above so does not require treatment at this stage, but the GP should continue to monitor her blood pressure
- In adults <60 years with stage 1 hypertension, consider starting antihypertensive drug treatment
- In adults >80 years with stage 1 hypertension, consider starting treatment if their clinic blood pressure is >150/90 mmHg

TIMEPOINT ⏱ 2

Two years later, Mrs Leigh moves house and registers with a new GP surgery. Her GP checks her blood pressure and again offers her ABPM, which she repeats. This time Mrs Leigh's average daytime ABPM is 158/99 mmHg. Mrs Leigh tells the GP that she has tried to improve her diet and exercise more, but she isn't sure that it has made much difference.

What treatment should the GP offer?

- Continue to encourage lifestyle changes
- Medication – step 1 treatment
  - Use an ACE inhibitor (ACEi, e.g. ramipril), angiotensin-II receptor blocker (ARB, e.g. losartan) or calcium channel blocker (CCB e.g. amlodipine)
  - The best option depends on the patient's age, whether or not they have type 2 diabetes, and whether they are of black African or African-Caribbean background
  - In this case the most appropriate option would be a CCB
  - A thiazide-like diuretic (TLD, e.g. indapamide) may be used instead of a CCB, if CCBs are not tolerated

What blood pressure target should the GP be aiming for?

- Clinic blood pressure targets
  - <140/90 mmHg if aged <80 years
  - <150/90 mmHg if aged ≥80 years
- ABPM/HBPM targets
  - <135/85 mmHg if aged <80 years
  - <145/85 mmHg if aged ≥80 years
- Be aware targets may be different if concurrent diabetes, renal or cardiovascular disease

The GP starts Mrs Leigh on 5 mg of amlodipine daily and promises to continue reviewing her blood pressure management.

TIMEPOINT ⏱ 3

One year later, Mrs Leigh has her blood pressure rechecked by the GP. She is happy with the amlodipine and does not think that she has had any side effects from it, but her clinic blood pressure is still 150/92 mmHg. Mrs Leigh asks the GP if she will need to start taking more tablets.

Which tablets could be added at this stage?

- ACE inhibitor (ACEi)
- Angiotensin-II receptor blocker (ARB)
- Thiazide-like diuretic (TLD)

If Mrs Leigh's blood pressure were to continue to worsen, an ACEi/ARB, CCB and TLD can all be used in combination. Ensure that the patient is compliant with the medication they have already been prescribed, and that they are taking it at the optimum dose.

What is resistant hypertension and what treatment can be given for this?

Resistant hypertension is hypertension not controlled in patients taking optimal doses of three drugs.

Management
- Confirm measurements with ABPM/HBPM
- Check for postural hypotension
- Check medication adherence
- A fourth drug can be added once the patient's serum potassium has been checked
  - If potassium ≤4.5 mmol/L, consider giving low-dose spironolactone
  - If potassium >4.5 mmol/L, consider giving an alpha or beta-blocker
- All patients with resistant hypertension should be referred to a specialist for advice

---

When should patients with hypertension be referred for same-day specialist review?

- If clinic blood pressure is ≥180/120 mmHg with any of:
  - Retinal haemorrhage
  - Papilloedema
  - New confusion
  - Chest pain
  - Signs of heart failure
  - Acute kidney injury
- If pheochromocytoma is suspected

TIMEPOINT 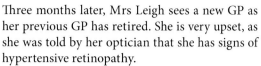 4

Three months later, Mrs Leigh sees a new GP as her previous GP has retired. She is very upset, as she was told by her optician that she has signs of hypertensive retinopathy.

She is angry that the previous GP had never told her about this or tested her for it. The new GP explains to Mrs Leigh about hypertensive retinopathy and how it can be treated. She reassures her that the most important part of managing hypertensive retinopathy is managing the underlying high blood pressure and that she will help her to do that.

Mrs Leigh accepts that part of the responsibility is hers, as in the past she has not always attended for blood pressure checks when invited, and she agrees to attend for more regular blood pressure checks in the future.

What are the signs of hypertensive retinopathy?

- Narrowing of arteries – 'copper' or 'silver' wiring
- Arteriovenous 'nipping' where arteries and veins cross
- Cotton wool spots – ischaemic swelling from blockages
- Superficial haemorrhages
- Exudates
- Papilloedema

How is hypertensive retinopathy managed?

- Manage hypertension
- Laser treatment
- Intravitreal injection of steroid or anti-VEGF

Case 7

TIMEPOINT 1

Mrs Written is a 74-year-old retired bookkeeper. She is a widow but has her best friend visit most days, except that her friend had gone away for a month on holiday. One day in July she presents to the A&E department after being found to be sleepy and less talkative than usual by her friend who had just returned.

Her past medical history includes type 2 diabetes mellitus, hypertension and dyslipidaemia.
She is currently taking atorvastatin, ramipril, amlodipine, indapamide and metformin.
She smokes 20 cigarettes/day – for the last 30 years – and usually drinks a bottle of wine with dinner each night.

On arrival in A&E, her observations are:

Respiratory rate: 17/min
Oxygen saturations: 99% on room air
Temperature: 36.7°C
Blood pressure: 150/80 mmHg
Heart rate: 80 bpm

Mrs Written responds to voice – V – on the AVPU scale. The remainder of the general examination is unremarkable except that she is slightly drowsy and somewhat inattentive to questions, appearing to be talking 'off topic' at times.

What initial investigations would need to be considered?

- Bloods – FBC, U&Es, LFTs, CRP, glucose
- CT head
- MRI head

Initial blood tests show the following:

Venous blood results

Sodium	103 mmol/L
Potassium	3.3 mmol/L
Urea	1.9 mmol/L
Creatinine	54 µmol/L
Haemoglobin	130 g/L
White cell count	7.0×10^9/L
Platelets	259×10^9/L
MCV	109 FL

CT head – involutional change consistent with age. Nil acute.

Key investigations in hyponatraemia

- Serum osmolality
- Urine osmolality
- Urine sodium
- Thyroid function tests
- 9 am cortisol
- Lipid profile
- Protein electrophoresis
- Glucose

How might Mrs Written be managed?

- The immediate management will involve attending to the severe hyponatraemia as the first priority. Mrs Written is neurologically compromised. However, the nature of the neurological state and its rate of change could not be ascertained. According to the level of sodium, efforts would be directed to improving the sodium level, avoiding factors

DOI: 10.1201/9781351257725-7

that could make it fall further and providing appropriate rates and forms of correction

- Hypertonic saline has been prescribed and given in this case; however, the rate of delivery of the initial 500 mL bag of 3% NaCl is not specified on the prescription
- Mrs Written currently takes indapamide which should be stopped

Common drugs associated with hyponatraemia

- Antidepressants: especially SSRIs
- Anti-epileptic medications: especially carbamazepine and sodium valproate
- Antidiuretic hormone analogues e.g. desmopressin, vasopressin, terlipressin
- Anticancer agents e.g. vincristine, cisplatin
- Anti-psychotic medications, e.g. haloperidol
- Diuretics, e.g. thiazides, indapamide,
- Proton-pump inhibitors, e.g. omeprazole

Mrs Written is noted to have a raised MCV. What might this indicate?

The causes are varied, but a raised MCV may be associated with chronic alcohol excess, which can have a direct impact on bone marrow function leading to an overall macrocytosis. Important causes of macrocytosis include B12 or folate deficiency, reticulocytosis and hypothyroidism.

TIMEPOINT 2

Eight hours later, repeat blood tests show the following:

Venous blood results

Sodium	130 mmol/L
Potassium	3.8 mmol/L
Urea	2.9 mmol/L
Creatinine	56 μmol/L

How much has the sodium risen in terms of mmol/hr?

It has risen by 27 mmol in 8 hours; therefore it has risen at a rate of over 3 mmol per hour.

TIMEPOINT 3

Four days later, it is noted by the nursing staff and the medical team that Mrs Written is now becoming persistently drowsy, and she seems to have reduced movement in her upper limbs.

Repeat U&Es show the following:

Venous blood results

Sodium	136 mmol/L
Potassium	3.9 mmol/L
Urea	2.8 mmol/L
Creatinine	54 μmol/L

This result shows an even further rise in serum sodium.

On examination, Mrs Written is inattentive, not responding to focused questions and had poor coordination of upper and lower limb movements.

What imaging investigations would be suitable to do?

- CT head
- MRI brain

The CT head comes back reported as normal; however, an MRI brain scan reveals likely pontine demyelination (Figure 7.1).

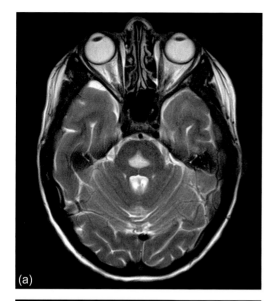

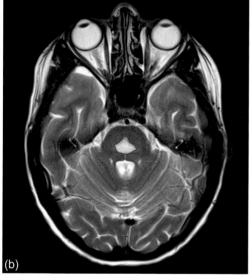

Figure 7.1 (a) Axial T2 magnetic resonance image through the brain. (b) The same image with demarcating abnormal high T2 signal within the pons (red outline). Given the patient's clinical presentation, imaging appearances would be in keeping with pontine myelinosis.

Mrs Written has developed central pontine demyelination (or osmotic demyelination) secondary to overly rapid correction of hyponatraemia. Other risk factors include alcoholism, malnutrition, liver disease, hypokalemia and long duration of hyponatraemia. An outline of recommended rates of correction is shown in Table 7.1.

Osmotic demyelination syndrome

Severe hypotonic hyponatraemia promotes the movement of water into the brain, and therefore in very acute cases, can cause cerebral oedema. However, over time, the brain is able to adapt and reduce cerebral volume to minimise the complications and oedema. Cerebral adaptation to hyponatraemia occurs after 2–3 days. After this time, osmotic demyelination syndrome can occur when severe hyponatraemia is corrected too rapidly and the brain volume begins to shrink. The exact mechanism for this is not fully understood. Osmotic demyelination syndrome presents in a biphasic pattern, showing initial improvement in symptoms, followed by new neurological signs. These can include progressive quadriplegia, ophthalmoplegia, seizures, behavioural abnormalities and movement disorders. In very severe cases it can result in locked-in syndrome where patients lose the ability to move, speak or swallow. This is a result of demyelination of the central pons.

TIMEPOINT 🕐 4

Six months later, when visited by a distant cousin who lives in Australia, Mrs Written is now in a residential centre for patients with a range of neurological problems and has begun to regain upper limb movements with the help of physiotherapy.

Recent blood tests done by the local doctor show normal sodium levels. She has had many visits from her lifelong friend and is beginning to make new ones but finds it difficult to connect closely with people. She now drinks no alcohol and is served highly nutritious meals with vitamin B supplements.

Table 7.1 Rate of correction of hyponatraemia

Time from start of treatment	Management and therapeutic goal
Within first hour	• Manage in intensive care • Give a 100 mL bolus of 3% saline IV up to 3 times • Aim to increase plasma sodium concentration by 4–6 mmol/L in the first 6 hours
Subsequent	• Start a slow IV infusion of 0.9% saline • Aim to start treatment for the underlying cause • Avoid increasing plasma sodium by >8 mmol/day • Recheck sodium levels at 6, 12, 24 and 48 hours

What is the overall prognosis of osmotic demyelination syndrome?

Prognosis is highly variable. Around 40–60% of patients seem to make a favourable level of neurological recovery, but there is around 5–15% mortality. The demyelination may be pontine, extrapontine or both and the symptoms usually correlate accordingly. Even in more severe cases that require ventilatory support, it is possible to make full functional recovery.

Prognosis appears to have improved in recent decades. This may be due to several factors, including earlier detection by MRI, current modern intensive care (such as precision fluid and electrolyte management) and improved pathophysiological understanding. In addition, patients benefit from rapid initiation of rehabilitation.

FURTHER READING

1. Sterns RH. Disorders of plasma sodium – causes, consequences and correction. *NEJM* 2015. 372:55–65.
2. Sterns RH. Treatment of severe hyponatraemia. *Clin J Am Soc Nephrol* 2018. 13: 641–649.
3. Sterns RH. Evidence for managing hypernatraemia: is it just hyponatraemia in reverse? *Clin J Am Soc Nephrol* 2019. 14: 645–647.

Case 8

TIMEPOINT  1

Miss Denham is a 55-year-old artist who presented to the emergency department after coughing and feeling hot for 2 days. She has a diagnosis
of stage-IIIA serous ovarian cancer for which she
had a bilateral salpingo-oophorectomy and total
abdominal hysterectomy just over 2 months ago.
She was then started on paclitaxel and carbopla-
tin adjuvant chemotherapy, and finished her third
cycle 6 days ago. She was warned to seek medical
attention if she developed a fever or began to feel
unwell. Her sister visited and thought that she
seemed drowsy. She checked her temperature,
which was 38.7°C, and called an ambulance.

Prior to her cancer diagnosis she had no significant medical or surgical history. Her BMI is
34 and she smokes 20 cigarettes a day, but she has
never drunk any alcohol. She lives with her long-
term partner and has never had any children.

She is still sufficiently drowsy that no further
history can be taken in triage.

Her observations show:

Respiratory rate: 28/min
Oxygen saturations: 94% on room air
Temperature: 38.6°C
Blood pressure: 96/66 mmHg
Heart rate: 105 bpm

The nurse calculates that the NEWS score is 8 and
calls the doctor for an urgent review.

> A NEWS score of >5 should always
> prompt a sepsis screen including a check
> for red flags.

What are the red flags for sepsis, according to the UK Sepsis Trust?

- V/P/U on AVPU
- Acutely confused
- Systolic BP ≤90 mmHg, or a drop of >40
  from the patient's usual systolic average
- Heart rate >130 bpm
- RR ≥25/min
- Requiring oxygen to saturate ≥92%
- Non-blanching rash, mottled, ashen or
  cyanotic
- Anuric for 18 hours or urine output
  <0.5 mL/kg/hour
- Lactate ≥2 mmol/L
- Recent chemotherapy

> Sepsis amber flags include immunosup-
> pression, temperature <36°C, signs of
> wound or skin infection, recent surgery or
> trauma.

What is your initial management of Miss Denham?

The Sepsis 6 protocol should be initiated as a matter of priority.

1. Give oxygen to keep saturations above 94%
2. Take blood cultures
   i. At this stage, blood tests should be sent to
      include a full blood count, urea and elec-
      trolytes, liver function tests, C reactive
      protein and a coagulation screen. It may
      also be appropriate to send a blood film

ii. As well as blood cultures, cultures should be taken from any other possible sources of infection, including urine, sputum, stool, skin/wound and any vascular lines/ports
3. Give intravenous antibiotics
    i. These should be given according to local guidelines for neutropenic sepsis, with guidance from the microbiology team if required. A typical regime may be
        i. Tazocin (piperacillin-tazobactam) 4.5 g IV QDS
        ii. Add in vancomycin if MRSA colonised
        iii. Add in a STAT dose of gentamicin if hypotensive despite fluid resuscitation
        iv. If penicillin allergic, give meropenem or if patient has anaphylaxis to penicillin, give vancomycin, gentamicin and metronidazole
        v. If treating a pneumonia, consider covering for atypical microorganisms with a macrolide
4. Give an intravenous fluid challenge
5. Measure the serum lactate (a blood gas may be used to check a point of care measurement)
6. Measure urine output with a urometer

A systems examination should then be conducted to establish a possible infective source, including:

- Cardiovascular: endocarditis
- Respiratory and chest X-ray: pneumonia
- Rashes and wounds: cellulitis, skin infection or meningitis
- Joints: septic arthritis
- Ears: otitis media
- Neurological: meningitis, encephalitis
- Abdominal and urine dip: gastroenteritis, cholecystitis, cholangitis, pancreatitis, urinary tract infection or pyelonephritis

Miss Denham's initial blood tests showed the following:

Venous blood results

Haemoglobin	98 g/L
White cell count	1.2×10^9/L
Neutrophils	0.4×10^9/L
Platelets	120×10^9/L
CRP	93 mg/L

Her observations are repeated and show:

Respiratory rate: 24/min
Oxygen saturations: 99% on 2 litres of oxygen
Temperature: 38.9°C
Blood pressure: 111/78 mmHg
Heart rate: 98 bpm

Definition of febrile neutropenia

Oral temperature ≥ 38.5°C or two consecutive readings of ≥ 38.0°C 1 hour apart, plus neutrophils $\leq 0.5 \times 10^9$/L.
    Be aware that paracetamol and steroids may mask pyrexia – if the patient appears unwell, consider sepsis.

What are the causes of neutropenia?

Moderate neutropenia is defined as neutrophils $0.5–1.0 \times 10^9$/L.
    Severe neutropenia is defined as neutrophils $<0.5 \times 10^9$/L.
    There are many causes of neutropenia aside from recent chemotherapy, including:

- Infection – EBV, CMV, HIV, hepatitis B, hepatitis C, typhoid, malaria, measles, dengue fever, toxoplasmosis
- Autoimmune
- Thyroid dysfunction
- Malignant bone marrow infiltration
- Aplastic anaemia
- B12/folate/iron deficiency
- Radiotherapy
- Drugs and chemical agents: chloramphenicol, alcohol, phenytoin, benzene, organophosphates
- Hypersplenism
- Felty's syndrome (rheumatoid arthritis with splenomegaly and neutropenia)
- Rare congenital syndromes disrupting neutrophil production, e.g. Kostmann's syndrome, Chediak–Higashi, X-linked agammaglobulinaemia

TIMEPOINT ⏱ 2

Thirty-six hours later, Miss Denham is reviewed on the oncology ward. She has already received treatment according to the Sepsis 6 protocol, and was also started on G-CSF on the advice of the haematology team.

Her repeat blood tests show:

Venous blood results

Haemoglobin	102 g/L
White cell count	2.9×10^9/L
Neutrophils	1.5×10^9/L
Platelets	135×10^9/L
CRP	74 mg/L

What are the indications for and the common side effects of G-CSF?

There are four different versions of G-CSF currently available on the UK market: filgrastim, lenograstim, lipegfilgrastim and pegfilgrastim. They are given via subcutaneous injection, subcutaneous infusion or intravenous infusion.

Indications for G-CSF treatment:

- Reduction in duration of neutropenia and incidence of febrile neutropenia in cytotoxic chemotherapy of malignancy
- Reduction in duration of neutropenia in myeloablative therapy followed by bone marrow transplantation
- Reduction in the duration of neutropenia and associated complications following bone marrow or peripheral stem cell transplantation
- Mobilisation of peripheral blood progenitor cells for autologous infusion
- Mobilisation of peripheral blood progenitor cells in normal donors for allogeneic infusion
- Severe congenital neutropenia and history of severe or recurrent infections
- Severe cyclic neutropenia, or idiopathic neutropenia and history of severe or recurrent infections
- Persistent neutropenia in HIV infection

Common side effects of G-CSF treatment:

- Arthralgia
- Cutaneous vasculitis
- Dyspnoea
- Haemoptysis
- Headache
- Hypersensitivity
- Leucocytosis
- Pain
- Spleen abnormalities
- Thrombocytopenia

TIMEPOINT ⏱ 3

Two days later, the ward sister requests that Miss Denham is the first to be reviewed on the ward round as she has been unwell overnight. The sister reports that she has vomited four times overnight. She was reviewed by the night doctor who prescribed fluids and anti-emetics and did not escalate the situation any further.

On review during the ward round, Miss Denham reports that she still feels very nauseous and lethargic. She has severe cramping in her leg muscles and some paraesthesiae in her fingertips. She appears unwell.

Bloods taken on the phlebotomy round 2 hours earlier are reviewed and compared to bloods from the previous day (Table 8.1).

The doctor performs an arterial blood gas (Table 8.2).

An ECG is also done which demonstrates a long QT interval. There are no signs of hyperkalaemia on the ECG.

What is the most likely diagnosis to explain the sudden metabolic derangement?

Tumour lysis syndrome. This occurs when a very good response to treatment leads to the large release of intracellular contents into the circulation, leading to potentially dangerous metabolic derangement.

Table 8.1 Venous blood results

	Current bloods	Previous bloods
White cell count	4.9×10^9/L	3.7×10^9/L
Haemoglobin	113 g/L	107 g/L
Neutrophils	2.8×10^9/L	2.2×10^9/L
Platelets	193×10^9/L	168×10^9/L
Sodium	142 mmol/L	137 mmol/L
Potassium	6.2 mmol/L	5.1 mmol/L
Urea	8.7 mmol/L	4.9 mmol/L
Creatinine	124 µmol/L	72 µmol/L
Magnesium	0.52 mmol/L	0.91 mmol/L
Phosphate	2.3 mmol/L	1.2 mmol/L
Corrected calcium	1.84 mmol/L	2.22 mmol/L
Glucose	6.3 mmol/L	5.6 mmol/L
Urate	420 µmol/L	205 µmol/L

Table 8.2 Arterial blood gas results

pH	7.29
$PaCO_2$	4.2 kPa
PaO_2	12.3 kPa
HCO_3	15 mmol/L
Lactate	1.9 mmol/L
Sodium	136 mmol/L
Potassium	6.2 mmol/L
Chloride	106 mmol/L

> Tumour lysis syndrome occurs less commonly with solid tumours (the risk is much higher with haematological malignancy), but it is still a key differential diagnosis that must be ruled out in patients who are unwell post-chemotherapy.

It may lead to metabolic derangements including:

- Hyperkalaemia
- Hyperphosphataemia
- Secondary hypocalcaemia
- Hyperuricaemia (from protein metabolism)
- Acute kidney injury

Diagnosis is made according to the Cairo–Bishop criteria:

Laboratory tumour lysis syndrome
- $\geq$2 abnormal serum biochemistry results, in the same 24-hour period within 3 days prior to treatment until 7 days after starting treatment.
  - Urate $\geq$476 µmoL or >25% increase from baseline
  - Potassium $\geq$6.0 mmol/L or >25% increase from baseline
  - Phosphate $\geq$1.45 mmol/L or 25% increase from baseline
  - Calcium $\leq$1.75 mmol/L or 25% decrease from baseline

Clinical tumour lysis syndrome
- Acute kidney injury
- Arrhythmia
- Seizure, tetany or other symptomatic hypocalcaemia

Symptoms and signs may result from any of the metabolic abnormalities and include:

- Nausea and vomiting
- Diarrhoea
- Anorexia

- Lethargy
- Haematuria
- Heart failure
- Cardiac arrhythmias
- Seizures
- Muscle cramps
- Tetany
- Syncope
- Arthralgia
- Renal colic

What is the management of this situation, including that of the specific electrolyte abnormalities?

- Immediate resuscitation using an ABCDE approach
- Aggressive rehydration with intravenous fluids
- Start cardiac monitoring
- Investigations: check urea and electrolytes, magnesium, phosphate, parathyroid hormone, vitamin D levels and perform an ECG
- Treat specific electrolyte abnormalities
  - Hyperkalaemia
    - Restrict dietary potassium
    - Give intravenous fluids which do not contain potassium
    - Check the drug chart for causes of hyperkalaemia, e.g. NSAIDs, ACE inhibitors, angiotensin receptor blockers, potassium-sparing diuretics
    - Check the ECG for changes suggestive of hyperkalaemia, e.g.
      - Tall, tented T-waves
      - Flattened, widened, or absent P waves
      - Prolonged PR segment
      - Prolonged QRS interval
      - Potentially dangerous arrhythmias, e.g. junctional and ventricular escape rhythms, bundle branch or fascicular blocks
    - Calcium resonium 15 g PO OD-TDS may be suitable for mild cases
    - In moderate hyperkalaemia, give 10 units of fast-acting insulin with 50 mL of 50% dextrose, followed by a glucose 10% IV infusion 200–300 mL over 4 hours. BMs should be checked regularly
    - Nebulised salbutamol may also be given, 10–20 mg 2 hourly
    - In severe cases (K^+ ≥6.5 mmol/L, or with ECG changes), give 10 mL of 10% calcium gluconate IV. This can be repeated another two times after 10 minutes if needed. Be cautious if patient is taking digoxin
  - Hyperphosphataemia
    - Give 50 mL of 50% dextrose with 20 units of intravenous insulin
    - Phosphate binders may be required
  - Hypocalcaemia
    - Give 10 mmoL of 10% calcium gluconate via a slow IV infusion
    - Ideally calcium should not be given until phosphate is corrected
  - Hyperuricaemia
    - Loop diuretics such as furosemide may help to wash out excess urate
    - Rasburicase 200 microgram/kg by intravenous infusion, once daily for up to 7 days
- Once stable, electrolytes should be measured twice daily until resolution
- Renal replacement therapy may be necessary in severe cases

What prophylaxis can be given for tumour lysis syndrome?

- The main element of prophylaxis is aggressive hydration with intravenous fluids
  - 2–3 litres/m²/day are required
  - Patients should be monitored carefully due to the risk of fluid overload
  - Ideally, urine output should be maintained at over 100 mL/hour, with furosemide given if needed
- For high-risk patients, oral allopurinol may also be given
  - The dose varies from 100 to 900 mg daily, calculated according to their risk
- Rasburicase may also be given as prophylaxis

TIMEPOINT 🕐 4

Twelve days later, Miss Denham returns to the oncology clinic for an afternoon appointment. It is now 3 days since she was discharged from the ward. Blood tests taken that morning show the following:

Venous blood results

Haemoglobin	111 g/L
White cell count	6.3×10^9/L
Neutrophils	4.2×10^9/L
Platelets	203×10^9/L

She is informed that her white cell count has returned to normal, and the oncologist is keen for her to restart chemotherapy. However, Miss Denham is worried about becoming septic again and is increasingly concerned about other possible side effects of her chemotherapy.

What prophylaxis can be given to high-risk neutropenic patients?

Fluoroquinolone prophylaxis should be offered to patients during the expected period of neutropenia.

What are key side effects of chemotherapeutic agents to warn patients of?

This list is not comprehensive but covers some of the most common side effects of chemotherapy:

- Fatigue, breathlessness and dizziness secondary to anaemia
- Bruising, petechiae, bleeding mucosa, epistaxis
- Alopecia
- Palmar-plantar erythema
- Gastrointestinal complications, e.g. nausea, vomiting, diarrhoea, constipation, anorexia, heartburn, metallic taste, aphthous ulcers, weight loss
- Peripheral neuropathy
- Cognitive impairment
- Rashes
- Infection and sepsis
- Tinnitus

Patients may also require fertility counselling prior to commencing chemotherapy, and should receive information regarding the increased risk of thrombosis and renal damage.

Case 9

TIMEPOINT 🕐 1

Mrs Lock is a 62-year-old woman who took early retirement and now volunteers in a charity shop. She has felt a bit 'muzzy' in the head recently, finding it harder to read her favourite crime thrillers in the last few weeks and then over the last few days has developed an unpleasant headache, with some 'fuzziness' and double vision.

One day she was in the local post office; she'd forgotten to drink her usual two glasses of milk in the morning but felt it was really urgent to post a birthday card, despite the fact that the headache was worsening. It was a very hot day and she started to feel dizzy. Before reaching the counter, the other customers saw her sway to one side and then collapse and an ambulance was called.

Her past medical history includes hypertension and angina, which are both well-controlled. She takes diltiazem and ramipril.

She was taken to the emergency department and her observations were as follows:

Respiratory rate: 16/min
Oxygen saturations: 95% on room air
Temperature: 37.0°C
Blood pressure: 114/80 mmHg
Heart rate: 80 bpm

Examination revealed that Mrs Locke was pale looking, somewhat distracted and disorientated with evidence of visual disturbance with partial right CNVI and CNIII palsies.

CNII – impaired visual acuity
CNIII – right palsy
CNVI – partial right palsy

It was clear that Mrs Lock required admission to hospital and further assessment included a more detailed history and general physical examination.

What initial investigations would need to be done?

- Blood tests – including FBC, U&E, LFT, CRP, ESR, endocrine screen – TFTs, cortisol, FSH, LH, prolactin, IGF-1
- ECG
- CT head

Her blood results are shown in Table 9.1.

The CT head report was as follows: *There is a large mass in the pituitary fossa extending into the sphenoid sinus and laterally into the cavernous sinuses, within which there is a small focus of haemorrhage. There is complete erosion of the sella and the tumour bulges into the sphenoid and cavernous sinuses.*

What are the clinical priorities now?

- Establishment of cortisol and thyroxine status/replacement
- Ophthalmology review/opinion
- Neurosurgical opinion and further imaging via MRI

TIMEPOINT 🕐 2

The next day, Mrs Lock is now on an acute medical ward. She is taken for an MRI brain scan.

The MRI shows a pituitary macroadenoma with apoplexy, extending into the suprasellar cistern and right cavernous region.

Table 9.1 Venous blood results

White cell count	4.5×10^9/L	Corrected calcium	2.38 mmol/L
Haemoglobin	130 g/L	Albumin	31 g/L
Platelets	188×10^9/L	Bilirubin	21 μmol/L
CRP	2 mg/L	Alkaline phosphatase	173 U/L
Sodium	128 mmol/L	Alanine aminotransferase	43 U/L
Potassium	4.1 mmol/L	PT	11.2 secs
Urea	8.0 mmol/L	INR	1.0
Creatinine	61 μmol/L	APTT	17 secs
Magnesium	0.73 mmol/L	APTTR	1.0
Phosphate	0.81 mmol/L	ESR	87 mm/hr

Endocrine screen

Random cortisol [>350 nmol/L]	24 nmol/L	Prolactin [<700 mIU/L]	238 mIU/L
		IGF-1 [9–40 nmol/L]	7.6 nmol/L
FSH [Post-menopausal 25.8–134.8 IU/L]	1 IU/L	TSH [0.4–4.5 mU/L]	0.31 mU/L
LH [Post-menopausal 7.7–58.5 IU/L]	1.2 IU/L	T4 [12–22 pmol/L]	4.7 pmol/L

Mrs Lock's sister visited her on the ward and asked for an update on her condition. It was explained that:

- The preceding headache and visual disturbances followed by a collapse were all due to the same condition
- There is a (most likely benign) growth originating from the pituitary gland, with expansion to nearby structures, which has caused her symptoms; and a probable change to the situation today made the pituitary hormonal function suddenly reduced, leading to a lack of hormones that will need replacing
- In order to reduce the risk of further visual consequences and significant health problems, neurosurgical treatment is recommended

Mrs Lock is transferred to the regional neurosurgical centre. The tumour is removed endoscopically via a sphenoidotomy with wide clearance achieved.

Indications and complications of pituitary surgery

INDICATIONS

1. Pituitary apoplexy
2. Visual loss or field defects
3. Local cranial nerve palsies
4. Altered intracranial pressure
5. Altered level of consciousness

COMPLICATIONS

1. Altered pituitary function/diabetes insipidus
2. CSF rhinorrhoea
3. Anosmia
4. Nasal injury or perforation
5. Haemorrhage
6. Infection/meningitis
7. Incomplete resection

TIMEPOINT ⏲ 3

Six days later, 12 hours post-pituitary surgery, the ward-based clinical team follows local protocol in terms of using appropriate fluid management, initially intravenous and then oral hydrocortisone, followed by oral thyroxine to ensure adequate endocrine replacement therapy as part of a pituitary surgery 'post-operative' care bundle.

Mrs Lock is visited by an endocrine specialist nurse who gives important education about the need to be able to manage hydrocortisone replacement therapy.

What are the key educational issues for a patient initiating hydrocortisone replacement?

- Sick day rules (a regime for increasing hydrocortisone dosage when unwell, e.g. triple dosage for 48–72 hrs, followed by double dosage for the next 48–72 hrs)
- An emergency injection pack for intramuscular administration of 100 mg hydrocortisone if needed – with instructions in written or video format as how to perform this
- Websites with further information and self-help/patient support groups such as The Pituitary Foundation

Upon discharge, a copy of the inpatient summary with a date for a telephone support consultation and outpatient clinic were provided, and advice was given as to what to do if any of the recognised late complications of the operation were to take place.

TIMEPOINT ⏲ 4

Five weeks later, Mrs Lock is reassessed in endocrine clinic.

A cranial nerve examination is performed with the following findings:

CNI: mild reduced olfactory sensation since operation, but recovering.

CNII: not formally tested with Snellen chart. She reports normal far and near vision but ongoing significant diplopia. No visual field defect.
CNIII/IV/VI: full range of movement L eye. No abduction of R eye. No nystagmus or eye pain on movement. Mild right-sided ptosis.
CNV: normal sensory perception bilaterally in V1,2,3. Mild paraesthesia in R V1 ~0.5/10 in pain over R eyebrow.
CNVII: Full range of facial movement. No loss of taste.
CNVIII: Reports reduction in hearing in L ear. Normal hearing on whispering numbers.
CNIX/X/XI: No tongue fasciculations/weakness. No palatal/tongue deviation. Normal tongue movement and swallow (reported). Intact head turning and shoulder shrugging.

In conclusion: mild paraesthesia in R V1. R CNVI palsy. Mild R-sided ptosis.

A detailed discussion takes place between the consultant and Mrs Lock, covering the long-term aspects of pituitary replacement therapy; the planned regularity of endocrine clinic review; and the support that can be provided both from health professionals and support groups and online resources.

Overall, it is felt that reasonable recovery is being made and further follow-up with ophthalmology, endocrinology, the endocrine specialist nurse and both virtual and face-to-face MDT clinic reviews are booked.

What is cavernous sinus syndrome?

Cavernous sinus syndrome is when a lesion and/or vascular process causes impact on structures in the unilateral or bilateral cavernous sinuses; often causing cranial nerve palsies (Table 9.2).

Which cranial nerve palsies can occur in cavernous sinus syndrome?

Cranial nerves III (oculomotor), IV (trochlear), V1 (ophthalmic branch of trigeminal), V2 (maxillary branch of trigeminal) all run in a vertical line in the wall of the cavernous sinus. Cranial nerve VI (abducens) runs alongside the internal

Table 9.2 Causes of cranial nerve palsies

Cranial nerves	Clinical role	Clinical signs if altered	Aetiology of lesions
CNI	Smell	Impaired sense of smell	Cribriform plate invasion/injuries/infection; SOL; trauma; surgery
CNII	Vision	Visual problems – depending on location of lesion	Orbital disease; pituitary disease; vascular events/demyelination/SOL Separate pathologies affect acuity and visual fields
CNIII	Eye movements and role in eyelid function	Lowered eyelid and double vision	Posterior communicating artery aneurysm; nasopharyngeal carcinoma; Tolosa Hunt syndrome
CNIV	Eye movements	Double vision	Rare alone, often connected with CNIII palsy
CNV	Motor Sensory	Altered (one side) facial sensation	Mononeuritis; herpes zoster; trigeminal neuralgia; acoustic neuroma (esp. corneal reflex)
CNVI	Eye movements	Double vision	Trauma; raised ICP; Wernicke's encephalopathy; MS; mononeuritis multiplex
CNVII	Facial movements	Weak/absent facial muscles on affected side	UMN – CVA/SOL LMN – sarcoid; Bell's palsy; inner ear issues
CNVIII	Hearing and balance	Weak/absent hearing and altered balance on affected side	Acoustic neuroma; Paget's; local ear surgery/trauma
CNIX	Palatal function	Altered palatal function	Trauma; pathology in neck
CNX	Vagus nerve supply	Altered vagus function	Trauma; pathology in neck
CNXI	Supply to trapezius and sternocleidomastoid	Altered trapezius/sternocleidomastoid	Trauma; pathology in neck
CNXII	Supply to (one side) of tongue	Deviated tongue	Stroke; SOL; Bulbar palsy

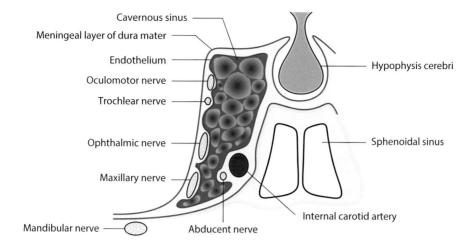

Cavernous sinus
Meningeal layer of dura mater
Endothelium
Oculomotor nerve
Trochlear nerve
Ophthalmic nerve
Maxillary nerve
Mandibular nerve
Abducent nerve
Hypophysis cerebri
Sphenoidal sinus
Internal carotid artery

Figure 9.1 Coronal section showing the relation of the cranial nerves to the cavernous sinus.

carotid artery in the medial wall, adjacent to the sphenoidal sinus. Therefore, lesions extending into the cavernous sinus can put pressure on any of these structures, causing cranial nerve palsies. See Figure 9.1.

What is the likelihood of recovery of the cranial nerve palsies?

Cranial nerve lesions when caused by temporary compression or reversible pathology can show a degree of recovery, often over months and often incomplete. Some cranial nerve lesions, if central to the pathological process of the (sometimes progressive) disease, may never recover.

FURTHER READING

1. Baldeweg, S.E. et al. 2016. Society for endocrinology endocrine emergency guidance: Emergency management of pituitary apoplexy in adult patients. *Endocrine Connections*. Available at: https://ec.bios cientifica.com/view/journals/ec/5/5/G12. xml

Case 10

TIMEPOINT 🕐 1

Mr Wood is a 17-year-old boy who has been brought to the emergency department after feeling wheezy. His mother, a local court magistrate, informs the medical team that her son had multiple episodes of bronchiolitis as an infant, severe eczema (especially as a young child) and hayfever symptoms every summer for the last few years. He has been playing rugby at school, but halfway through the game has had to stop due to feeling particularly wheezy. Initially, his chest just felt a bit tight, and he borrowed a friend's inhaler.

It is a cold day and he has a known history of asthma which was diagnosed in primary care, but he usually plays a lot of sports without a problem. He is currently studying for his A-levels and has been particularly stressed recently, and now frequently forgets to take his inhalers. After several puffs, his breathing is still worsening and an ambulance is called. When checked by the paramedics, his observations are:

Respiratory rate: 32/min
Oxygen saturations: 93% on room air
Temperature: 36.6°C
Blood pressure: 120/80 mmHg
Heart rate: 120 bpm

On examination, Mr Wood is noted to be a thin young man with remnant features of eczema on the flexural aspect of both upper arms. On auscultation of his chest there is widespread end-expiratory wheeze bilaterally.

Why is the finding of eczema important in this case?

Atopic dermatitis (eczema) in combination with asthma (as well as allergic rhinitis or hayfever) form part of a spectrum of IgE-mediated hypersensitivity disorders. These individuals also have an increased risk of IgE-mediated food allergies.

The peak expiratory flow rate (PEFR) is 220 L/min as performed by the paramedics. In the ambulance Mr Wood has two back-to-back salbutamol nebulisers. The paramedics are startled by the clear presence of severity features in this case, particularly given that Mr Wood had not experienced any critical care admissions nor previous hospitalisations at any time in the past (see Table 10.1 outlining stepwise descriptors of severity).

TIMEPOINT 🕐 2

Soon after his arrival at the emergency department a senior sister in emergency medicine obtains a peak flow reading and begins monitoring. She highlights the results to an emergency department doctor who requests that medical treatment be started immediately.

Initial PEFR in emergency department = 170 L/min (predicted 550 L/min = 31% of predicted).

What does the information obtained so far tell us about the severity of this episode?

Given his PEFR, Mr Wood is displaying signs of life-threatening asthma.

He had an ABG on admission which showed:

Arterial blood results

pH	7.4
$PaCO_2$	3.5 kPa
PaO_2	11.1 kPa

What does the blood gas tell us in acute asthma?

The pH is helpful as it might indicate acidosis, either respiratory or metabolic in origin. Low $PaCO_2$ is expected initially in asthma due to hyperventilation, but a rising or raised $PaCO_2$ (including

DOI: 10.1201/9781351257725-10

Table 10.1 Classification of acute asthma attacks

Moderate	Severe	Life-threatening
• Increasing symptoms • PEF >50–75% best or predicted • No features of acute severe asthma	Any one of: • PEF 33–50% best or predicted • Respiratory rate 25/min • Heart rate 110/min • Inability to complete sentences in one breath	In a patient with severe asthma any one of: • PEF <33% best or predicted • SpO_2 <92% • PaO_2 <8 kPa • Normal $PaCO_2$ (4.6–6.0 kPa) • Silent chest • Cyanosis • Poor respiratory effort • Arrhythmia • Exhaustion • Altered conscious level • Hypotension

within normal range) may indicate worsening of the clinical condition and/or the patient getting tired. The PaO_2 is important as a sufficient degree of oxygenation is essential for the patient.

Initial investigations show unremarkable venous blood tests. An ECG demonstrates sinus tachycardia. The chest X-ray shows evidence of hyperexpansion but no pneumothorax.

Mr Wood has treatment initiated including steroids, magnesium and regular nebulisers. Mr Wood is admitted after having been seen mid-afternoon by the duty respiratory consultant.

TIMEPOINT ⏱ 3

At 2 am (11 hours after admission), nurses monitoring Mr Wood's observations and peak flow on a regular basis feel concerned about his condition. After 5 hours on the ward, all Mr Wood's visitors have gone home and the nursing team has handed over to the night shift. Within another hour his condition seems to have worsened. It is now difficult for him to perform the peak flow test; values from the previous 2 hours have been falling, and a repeat blood gas is done by the ward cover doctor. This time the pH is 7.34, $PaCO_2$ 5.9 kPa and PaO_2 9.9 kPa. On the basis of these changes he urgently bleeps the medical registrar and, on her assessment, Mr Wood appears to be

tiring. Anaesthetists are called immediately and Mr Wood is intubated and taken to ITU.

Why did the blood gas result lead to such a clear set of clinical actions to be taken?

The key differences in this most recent blood gas are a fall in pH (even though only mildly below normal range) and rising $PaCO_2$. Whilst still within normal limits, the $PaCO_2$ has risen significantly compared to previous, showing relative hypoventilation, which is a concerning feature of asthma that needs prompt consideration of intubation and ventilation.

Mr Wood is in ITU for 4 days and then a general ward post-ITU for 3 more days. After a thorough respiratory nurse assessment pre-discharge and appropriate medication, Mr Wood is able to go home.

TIMEPOINT ⏱ 4

Three weeks later, Mr Wood is seen in the chest clinic. He has improved markedly from the period of admission and wishes to discuss whether to initiate further treatments in the future. The consultant, specialist nurse, Mr Wood and parents are all in the room. He is told that as a one-stop service, confirmatory tests are done in the clinic first visit to clarify the diagnostic certainty of asthma and then, if confirmed, there is a stepwise incremental approach to the next levels of treatment and a range of preventative strategies for maintaining wellbeing where possible. Those include:

- Avoidance of triggers (such as cats/dogs/passive smoking/high pollution areas, etc.)
- Obtaining of annual influenza and pneumococcal vaccination

The consultant in clinic discusses a wide range of categories of treatment of asthma, including the various forms of inhalers and nebulised treatment, and then mentions oral options including occasional need for prednisolone, montelukast and the newest treatment options.

Mr Wood's mother asks specifically about two medications that she read about in the newspaper.

What are montelukast and omalizumab?

Montelukast is a leukotriene receptor antagonist.

Omalizumab is a medicine which provides a monoclonal antibody against IgE, given as a subcutaneous injection every 4 weeks.

What are the factors making omalizumab more likely to be a successful treatment?

The British National Formulary clearly suggests that omalizumab should be considered under the following circumstances after a full trial of standard therapy:

'Optimised standard therapy is defined as a full trial of and, if tolerated, documented compliance with inhaled high-dose corticosteroids, long-acting beta-2 agonists, leukotriene receptor antagonists, theophyllines, oral corticosteroids, and smoking cessation if clinically appropriate'.

The means of clarifying the dose is through adjustment via IgE level and body weight.

Mr Wood then has a combined investigation protocol in the clinic, comprising blood tests, chest X-ray and spirometry.

What is spirometry?

Spirometry is a core element of lung function tests. Alongside spirometry (whether pre- or post-bronchodilator), other key lung function tests include flow volume loops and transfer factor (diffusion capacity). It is very helpful diagnostically given the subcategories of results available. The central spirometry measures include the forced expiratory volume able to be produced in 1 second (FEV1) and the overall forced vital capacity measurement (FVC) – the complete exhaled volume. The proportion that arises from dividing the value of FEV1 by FVC gives data to indicate whether the patient has a normal status, restrictive lung condition or obstructive lung condition. In restrictive conditions, the proportion of FEV1/FVC may be normal, giving a value of 0.7 or above. In obstructive conditions, which include asthma and chronic obstructive pulmonary disease (COPD), the result would usually be reduced.

Asthma, unlike some other conditions, should have a degree of bronchodilator responsivity – thus it would be expected to show 15–20% improvement via repeated spirometry. In some patients with asthma, the repeat spirometry post-bronchodilator can return values back to within normal range. Non-reversibility does not completely exclude asthma, but the continuum and spectrum of asthma and COPD especially in people older than teenagers is not clear-cut.

FURTHER READING

1. BTS/SIGN British Guideline on the Management of Asthma. Available at: www.brit-thoracic.org.uk/quality-improvement/guidelines/asthma/

Case 11

TIMEPOINT 🕐 1

Mrs Matt is a 72-year-old woman who loves walking breaks and family outings with her niece and nephew. Over the course of 3 days after a hill-walking holiday, she felt more tired than usual, a sense of feeling 'hot and bothered' and did not feel like socialising. This worsened to feeling muzzy-headed and the need to stay in bed. Her best friend came to see her and was shocked and concerned to find her exhibiting confusion and drowsiness, and therefore called for an ambulance.

She normally lives alone and just has a past history of chronic sinusitis. She has no medication allergies and no regular medicines. She only drinks alcohol occasionally with friends and does not smoke.

On arrival at the emergency department, the team assesses her condition urgently. Observations are as follows:

Respiratory rate: 25/min
Oxygen saturations: 96% on room air
Temperature: 37.8°C
Blood pressure: 110/70 mmHg
Heart rate: 89 bpm

On initial examination, her response is P (pain) on the AVPU scale and GCS 10/15 (E 4 M 4 V 2).

Urgent intravenous access is obtained, and routine blood tests and cultures taken. Intravenous paracetamol is given for a low-grade fever.

There is no obvious unilateral weakness. Capillary glucose is 6.9 mmol/L.

Given Mrs Matt's fever, confusion, and altered GCS, an urgent CT brain scan is requested and treatment with IV ceftriaxone and aciclovir is initiated.

See Table 11.1 for the laboratory blood test results.

What are the differential diagnoses at this stage and what investigations would help to confirm or exclude these?

The management of Mrs Matt thus far would suggest initial consideration of meningitis or encephalitis as leading differentials. Other possible causes of fever, confusion and altered consciousness often depend on the context, location and immunocompetency of the patient. Other broad differentials thus to be borne in mind would include atypical presentation of other forms of bacterial sepsis; cerebral vascular events (including subarachnoid haemorrhage or venous sinus thrombosis); cerebral vasculitis; and other infections such as CNS TB, CMV, cerebral malaria and leptospirosis.

TIMEPOINT 🕐 2

Three hours later, observations are as follows:

Respiratory rate: 25/min
Oxygen saturations: 96% on room air
Temperature: 37.5°C
Blood pressure: 120/70 mmHg
Heart rate: 82 bpm

Mrs Matt has had her CT brain scan but is awaiting the formal report. Mrs Matt's friend is with her and is told that if the CT scan is normal, the next important investigation to perform is a lumbar puncture. Although Mrs Matt is too confused to give formal informed consent for this procedure, the correct documentation is completed to confirm that the procedure is in Mrs Matt's best interests and there are no differences in opinion amongst the nursing team, medical team or close friend on that topic.

Table 11.1 Venous blood results

White cell count	12.3 × 10⁹/L	Corrected calcium	2.20 mmol/L
Haemoglobin	102 g/L	Albumin	32 g/L
Platelets	167 × 10⁹/L	Bilirubin	23 μmol/L
CRP	4 mg/L	Alkaline phosphatase	120 U/L
Sodium	137 mmol/L	Alanine aminotransferase	45U/L
Potassium	4.2 mmol/L	PT	11.4 secs
Urea	4.2 mmol/L	INR	1.0
Creatinine	62 μmol/L	APTT	17 secs
Magnesium	0.76 mmol/L	APTTR	1.0
Phosphate	0.83 mmol/L	ESR	98 mm/hr

A short while later, all the results currently available are reviewed by the admitting medical consultant. Mrs Matt's GCS has improved to 14/15.

The CT scan is normal.

The LP result shows a mildly raised lymphocyte count and protein. HSV culture results from the CSF are still awaited. The overall context leads to ongoing treatment to be continued with a plan for an MRI brain.

The attending consultant asks her team the indications for and interpretation of a lumbar puncture. See Table 11.2.

Mrs Matt goes on to have an MRI brain scan.

Indications and interpretation of a lumbar puncture

A lumbar puncture is a procedure regularly undertaken for diagnostic purposes especially in acutely unwell patients with the main indications being for assisting in the diagnosis of any form of meningo-encephalitis; subarachnoid haemorrhage, multiple sclerosis and a variety of other inflammatory and neoplastic neurological disorders. Please see Table 11.2.

The indications need to be clear and the contraindications include raised intracranial pressure and significant bleeding tendency.

A sample of clear colourless CSF is obtained (when normal).

It can be sent for a wide range of investigations; in this case it was sent for the following:

- Microscopy (WCC & RCC), culture and sensitivity
- Protein
- Glucose
- Cytology
- HSV PCR
- Other viral PCR

In cases where subarachnoid haemorrhage is suspected, a sample should be sent for xanthochromia. In this instance, LP should not be done until at least 12 hours have passed since the onset of headache.

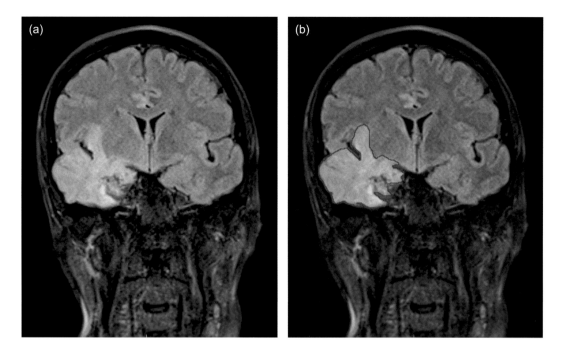

Figure 11.1 (a) MRI fluid attenuation inversion recovery (FLAIR) coronal image and (b) red outline on the same FLAIR image demarcates abnormal cortical and subcortical high signal in the right temporal lobe.

Table 11.2 Lumbar puncture result interpretation

	Normal	Bacterial	Viral	HSV encephalitis	SAH
Opening pressure (cmH$_2$O)	7–20	Often +++	Normal or slight +	Normal or slight +	Often +/++
Appearance	Clear	Purulent	Clear	Clear	May be clear/ reddish
Protein (g/L)	0.18–0.45	>1	<1	0.5–1	>0.45
Glucose (mmol/L)	60% or more of blood value	<60% of blood value	60% or more of blood value	60% or more of blood value	60% or more of blood value
Bacterial culture	Negative	60–90% positive	Negative	Negative	Negative
White cell count (mm^3)	<3	>500 – mostly neutrophils	<1000 – mostly lymphocytes	<1000 – mostly lymphocytes	Normal
Red cell count (mm^3)	<5	<5	+/–	+	High+++/ xanthochromia
HSV PCR	Negative	Negative	Negative	Positive	Negative

The MRI scan shows typical features of HSV encephalitis. See Figure 11.1.

What does a CT brain typically show in HSV encephalitis?

CT scanning may show low-density altered appearances in the temporal and/or frontal regions but will most often be reported as normal.

What does MRI typically show in HSV encephalitis?

MRI is the gold standard imaging modality for this condition and is abnormal in around 90% of cases; it is relevant to note that this percentage is much lower in other subtypes of encephalitis such as autoimmune. It will generally show marked temporal lobe changes and/or frontal lobe features and in addition basal ganglia and thalamic alterations may be observed.

With herpes simplex encephalitis, changes typically occur within the anterior and medial aspects of the temporal lobes. Similar high signal will be seen on T2 and isotropic images – diffusion-weighted imaging (DWI) – with corresponding abnormally low apparent diffusion coefficient (ADC) values or 'abnormal restricted diffusion'. There will be varying patterns of enhancement after contrast administration.

What are the causes of encephalitis other than HSV?

OTHER VIRAL CAUSES

- Varicella
- Enterovirus
- Japanese encephalitis
- West Nile virus (an arboviral type)
- Saint Louis encephalitis
- CMV
- Subacute sclerosing panencephalitis (SSPE) – caused by measles virus

AUTOIMMUNE ENCEPHALITIS

Autoimmune encephalitis is an increasingly recognised non-infective form of encephalitis that may present to both physical and psychiatric medical services. A range of antibody and

CSF-based diagnostics are still in development with improving recognition amongst specialists in the field.

TIMEPOINT ⏱ 3

On day 3, observations are as follows:

Respiratory rate: 25/min
Oxygen saturations: 96% on room air
Temperature: 37.1°C
Blood pressure: 140/80 mmHg
Heart rate: 72 bpm

Mrs Matt's GCS is 14/15 due to ongoing disorientation.

The CSF HSV PCR result comes back positive.

Therefore, the diagnosis of HSV encephalitis is made.

What should be done about the ceftriaxone and aciclovir?

Most international recommendations for ongoing HSV encephalitis treatment recommend a 14–21-day course of IV aciclovir – without need for antibiotics when confirmed as such.

The predictors of outcome relate to the degree of severity of illness on admission and various other clinical factors. Factors favouring poorer outcomes include the following: delay in initiating aciclovir treatment; GCS <8 on arrival; an age of 65 or over and a requirement for admission to critical care.

Are there any other tests that could be considered?

In order of increasing complexity, tests that can be worth considering are:

- HIV test
- EEG
- In cases of diagnostic uncertainty, a brain biopsy can be done to give a definitive tissue diagnosis. The brain biopsy in HSV encephalitis can show nuclei with a ground glass appearance as a result of viral particle accumulation. *Cowdry* bodies (type A) which are

surrounded by a clear halo with chromatin margination are also a characteristic finding

TIMEPOINT ⏱ 4

On day 120, Mrs Matt is now in a residential neuro-rehabilitation centre.

Her observations are as follows:

Respiratory rate: 25/min
Oxygen saturations: 96% on room air
Temperature: 37.0°C
Blood pressure: 137/81 mmHg
Heart rate: 72 bpm

Mrs Matt is able to swallow but her speech is still altered; she has a slow irregular gait. She is visited daily by family and friends who regularly participate in multidisciplinary meetings and receive written update reports from physiotherapy, occupational therapy, speech and language therapy and the clinical psychologist. It is common in the post-encephalitis setting to find a very significant change in personality, memory and higher cognitive functioning, which is often amenable to intensive neuro-rehabilitation. Mrs Matt continues to receive neuro-rehabilitation for many months.

What is the clinical outcome of HSV encephalitis?

The condition has a high mortality if untreated. Where managed appropriately, a proportion will need critical care management, including intubation and ventilation (e.g. 10–20%), and some will have seizures. Estimates suggest 40–50% of patients will have near-complete neurological recovery at 1 year, meaning most patients will have some form of neuropsychological impact long term.

FURTHER READING

1. www.clinmed.rcpjournal.org/content/18/2/155.full.pdf
2. www.nejm.org/doi/full/10.1056/NEJMra1708714
3. https://ccforum.biomedcentral.com/articles/10.1186/s13054-015-1046-y

Case 12

TIMEPOINT 1

Mr Hamilton is a 44-year-old builder who attends the emergency department complaining of severe back pain. His wife is more concerned about the fact that he has become increasingly unsteady on his feet over the last few days, to the point where he is now using her for support.

He reports that the pain started around 3 days ago in his lower back and has been gradually worsening. The pain is equal on both sides and worse on movement, and not improved by simple analgesia. He struggles to describe exactly what the pain feels like although he does mention that he is getting shooting and tingling pains down both legs. He agrees that his walking has been a little wobbly since the pain started, but he assumed it was just because the pain was so bad. When the emergency department doctor asks directly, Mr Hamilton admits that he had a single episode of urinary incontinence last night. He adds that he has been unusually constipated this week despite not making any changes to his diet.

He is usually fit and well, although he has just recovered from a nasty bout of 'flu' which left him in bed for a few days 2 weeks back. He had an appendicectomy at age 17 but has not had any other operations. He doesn't take any regular medications but is allergic to codeine. He drinks 4–5 pints of lager at the pub with his colleagues each Friday night but not much outside of that. He smokes 15 cigarettes a day and is proud of having cut down from 20 over the last year. He is still aiming to cut down further if he can to set a good example for his children. His father died at 63 of a heart attack, and his mother is alive and well. He doesn't have any other specific family history that he is aware of.

His observations are:

Respiratory rate: 18/min
Oxygen saturations: 98% on room air
Temperature: 35.7°C
Blood pressure lying: 127/94 mmHg
Blood pressure standing: 103/72 mmHg
Heart rate: 89 bpm

The routine panel of blood tests sent by the emergency department triage is normal.

Cardiovascular, respiratory, abdominal and cranial nerve examinations are unremarkable. There is no obvious abnormality on inspection of the back and legs, and the alignment of the spine appears normal. There is no tenderness to palpation of the spinous processes, paraspinal musculature or any other parts of the back. All passive and active movements of the spine are within normal limits. Schober's test is normal. There are no abnormalities on upper limb neurological examination.

On examination of the lower limbs, tone appears reduced throughout. Power is significantly reduced in ankle dorsiflexion, plantarflexion, inversion and eversion, as well as flexion and extension at the knee. All defects are equal bilaterally. Power of the hip movements is normal. Knee and ankle jerks are absent bilaterally. Flexion of the toes is observed on testing of the Babinski sign. Sensation to light touch is normal in all dermatomes. Coordination is poor on all tests conducted and gait appears ataxic in nature. Romberg's test is negative.

The emergency department doctor is concerned about the findings of his neurological examination and phones the neurology team to ask them to review Mr Hamilton. The neurology

Table 12.1 Upper vs. lower motor neuron signs

Upper motor neuron signs	Lower motor neuron signs
Pronator drift	Wasting and fasciculation
Increased tone +/– ankle clonus	Decreased or normal tone
Brisk reflexes	Reduced or absent reflexes
Positive (extensor) Babinski	Normal (flexor) Babinski
Pyramidal weakness	Differing patterns of weakness according to cause

registrar agrees that the findings are concerning and promises to review Mr Hamilton by the end of the day (Table 12.1).

What are the differential diagnoses for peripheral neuropathy?

- Metabolic
  - Diabetes mellitus and hypoglycaemia
  - Renal failure
  - Hypothyroidism
- Vasculitides and chronic vascular ischaemic disease
- Malignancies and paraneoplastic syndromes
- Inflammatory
  - Guillain–Barré syndrome
  - Sarcoidosis
- Infections
  - Leprosy
  - HIV
  - Syphilis
  - Lyme disease
  - Tetanus
  - Diphtheria
- Nutritional
  - Alcoholic excess
  - Low thiamine, vitamin B12 or folate
- Heavy metal poisoning
  - Mercury
  - Lead
  - Arsenic
- Congenital
  - Charcot–Marie–Tooth disease
  - Friedreich's ataxia
  - Porphyria
- Drugs
  - Phenytoin
  - Nitrofurantoin
  - Isoniazid
  - Vincristine
  - Gold
  - Cisplastin
  - Metronidazole

What signs and symptoms are typically associated with autonomic dysfunction and how may these be tested?

Symptoms and signs of autonomic dysfunction:

- Postural hypotension with or without syncope
- Anhidrosis or hyperhidrosis
- Hypothermia and hyperthermia
- Visual issues such as blurred vision, difficulty focusing, reduced lacrimation and abnormal pupillary reflexes
- Ejaculatory failure and erectile dysfunction
- Urinary incontinence or retention
- Tachy- and bradyarrhythmias
- Gastrointestinal issues such as constipation, diarrhoea, gastroparesis, dry mouth and fecal incontinence
- Horner's syndrome
- Holmes–Adie syndrome

Methods of testing for autonomic dysfunction:

- Secondary care
  - Lying/standing blood pressure
  - Urodynamics and cystometry
  - Assessment of gastroparesis via barium swallows, gastric emptying scintigraphy testing, capsule testing or endoscopy
- Specialist
  - Deep breathing test to assess vagal function. Heart rate is monitored throughout the testing to assess whether the patient has lost their physiological respiratory sinus arrhythmia
  - Valsalva manoeuvres to assess vagal function and adrenergic response. Blood pressure and heart rate are monitored during the manoeuvre
  - Tilt table testing to assess adrenergic response. The tilt table is used to create orthostatic stress. Blood pressure, heart rate and symptoms are monitored throughout the testing
  - Quantitative sudomotor axon reflex testing to assess sympathetic cholinergic function. This uses a special device to assess the rate and volume of sweating

TIMEPOINT ⏱ 2

Three hours later, the neurology registrar arrives to review Mr Hamilton. She reviews the history and examination of the emergency department doctor and is concerned about the possibility of Guillain–Barré syndrome, in light of an acute bilateral lower motor neuron peripheral neuropathy with a history of a recent viral infection. She is keen to send him for some further tests.

Key point

Guillain–Barré syndrome classically occurs 1–3 weeks after a respiratory or gastrointestinal infection
  Important causes include:

- *Campylobacter jejuni*
- Cytomegalovirus
- Epstein–Barr Virus
- *Haemophilus influenzae*
- Hepatitis A, B, C and E
- HIV
- Influenza virus
- *Mycoplasma pneumoniae*
- Zika virus

What investigations might be carried out at this stage?

Although Guillain–Barré syndrome is a clinical diagnosis, there are supportive tests which may be useful.

- Lumbar puncture shows high protein levels with normal cell counts. This is known as cytoalbuminaemic dissociation
- Repeated spirometry is required to assess for deterioration in lung function
- Nerve conduction studies are abnormal in 85% of patients
- Testing for antiganglioside antibodies: anti-GM1, anti-GD1b, anti-GT1a, anti-GD1a and anti-GQ1b may all be positive. There is some evidence to suggest that different antibodies are associated with different subtypes of the disease and may reflect prognosis

What are the typical features that you would expect to see on nerve conduction studies?

Nerve conduction studies are useful in that they might allow you to distinguish between demyelinating and axonal neuropathies. Studies can also suggest whether the syndrome is likely to be hereditary or acquired.

Typical features of a demyelinating neuropathy are:

- Prolonged F-wave latency
- Prolonged distal motor latency
- Reduced motor neuron conduction velocity
- Increased temporal dispersion
- Focal conduction blocks

Studies may be normal at first presentation and may need to be repeated after around 2 weeks for accurate results.

What is the management of Guillain–Barré syndrome?

Guillain–Barré syndrome is the most common cause of acute neuromuscular paralysis, so it is important to be aware of the basic elements of management.

- Supportive care
  - Pressure care
  - Venous thromboembolic prophylaxis
  - Speech and language input as speech and swallow may be affected
  - Close monitoring of respiratory function (may require intensive care input)
  - Cardiac and haemodynamic monitoring due to likely autonomic dysfunction
  - Bowel and bladder care as required
  - Psychological input: many patients become depressed due to the sudden disability
  - Physiotherapy and rehabilitation
- Therapeutic
  - Plasma exchange – a usual regime is five sessions over 2 weeks
  - Intravenous immunoglobulin (IVIg)
    - 0.4 g/kg daily for 5 days if unable to walk unaided
    - Most effective if used within 2 weeks from onset of weakness
  - May require more than one course
  - No evidence for steroids

The neurology registrar discusses the cases with her consultant who agrees that Mr Hamilton should be admitted to the neurology ward for a course of intravenous immunoglobulin.

TIMEPOINT 🕐 3

Five days later, the junior doctor covering the neurology ward is called to see Mr Hamilton as his latest observations have been scoring on the NEWS chart.

His observations are:

Respiratory rate: 27/min
Oxygen saturations: 84% on room air
Temperature: 35.4°C
Blood pressure: 135/87 mmHg
Heart rate: 124 bpm

The junior doctor asks Mr Hamilton how he is feeling and he replies that he is feeling very breathless. He is struggling to complete full sentences and does not appear to be orientated to time, place or person.

On examination his chest sounds clear, but he is requiring the use of accessory muscles of

Table 12.2 Spirometry results

	Spirometry results for Mr Hamilton from today	Predicted value for demographic
FVC	2.12 L	5.50 L
FEV1	1.67 L	4.35 L
FEV1/FVC	0.79	0.80

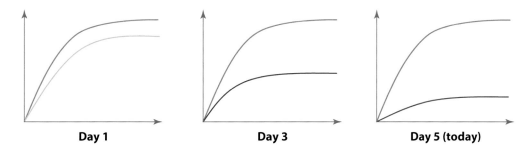

Figure 12.1 Spirometry graphs for Mr Hamilton. Mr Hamilton is a 44-year-old Caucasian male who is 182 cm tall. He weighs 77 kg. Graph demonstrates spirometry with the x-axis showing time, and the y-axis showing lung volume. Green lines show the predicted values for a patient of Mr Hamilton's demographic. Reference values from https://vitalograph.co.uk/resources/gli-normal-values.

ventilation and despite this has reduced chest expansion. The junior doctor is very concerned about the evidence of respiratory distress. She starts him on high-flow oxygen and quickly checks the spirometry results from today (Table 12.2). She realises that somehow the results have been missed, and they have not been reviewed by a senior member of the team. She calls the critical care outreach team and bleeps her registrar to attend urgently. The registrar arrives after a couple of minutes and asks the junior doctor to perform an ABG now so that it will be ready for when the critical care outreach team arrives. By this time Mr Hamilton has been on 15 litres of oxygen for around 5 minutes.

What does the spirometry demonstrate? What might this represent in the context of his likely diagnosis?

The spirometry demonstrates a reduced FEV1 and reduced FVC, both of which are less than 80% of the predicted value for Mr Hamilton's demographic. The ratio is still greater than 70%

of the predicted value (normal). This would be in keeping with a restrictive defect, which would be the expected pattern in a patient with respiratory distress caused by neuromuscular weakness. The weakness leads to insufficient ventilation which will eventually manifest as respiratory distress.

The graphs also suggest a worsening restrictive defect which would be in keeping with progressive weakness of the respiratory muscles related to his diagnosis of Guillain–Barré syndrome. See Figure 12.1.

Studies suggest that invasive ventilation is likely to be required when the vital capacity falls below 20 mL/kg (equivalent to less than 1.54 L in Mr Hamilton).

The junior doctor returns to Mr Hamilton's bedside with the ABG reading and shows it to the critical care outreach team which has just arrived on the ward (Table 12.3).

What does the ABG show?

The arterial blood gas shows a type 2 (hypercapnic) respiratory failure. This is a respiratory acidosis caused by carbon dioxide being retained secondary to hypoventilation (as a result of neuromuscular paralysis of the respiratory muscles).

The critical care outreach team feels that Mr Hamilton's respiratory status has deteriorated to the point where he will need non-invasive and possibly invasive ventilation, so he is transferred to the intensive care unit for stabilization.

He remains there for 3 weeks before being stepped back down to the general medical ward.

Table 12.3 Arterial blood gas results

pH	7.19
PCO_2	7.9 kPa
PO_2	6.4 kPa
HCO_3	21.9 mmol/L
Base excess	–5.3 mmol/L
Lactate	1.8 mmol/L

After 5 weeks in hospital he is discharged to a rehabilitation facility for 2 weeks, and then finally to his own home with ongoing input from community physiotherapists and occupational therapy.

TIMEPOINT ⏱ 4

Six weeks after his discharge home, Mr Hamilton attends a follow-up outpatient appointment in the neurology clinic with his wife.

His gait is now normal and he has regained his previous bladder, bowel and respiratory function. However, he is concerned about the fact that he continues to have lower back pain with shooting pains down his legs. He describes having intermittent 'electric shock' sensations and occasionally gets pins and needles.

The neurologist explains that this sounds like neuropathic pain which is a common complication of Guillain–Barré syndrome.

What are the causes of neuropathic pain?

Central causes

- Stroke
- Multiple sclerosis
- Spinal cord injury

Technically, any peripheral neuropathy can cause neuropathic pain. However, common peripheral causes include:

- Diabetic neuropathy
- Postherpetic neuralgia
- Trigeminal neuralgia
- Post-infective neuropathy (such as Guillain–Barré syndrome)
- Alcoholic neuropathy (secondary to vitamin B1 deficiency)
- Post-operative scar pain

- Post-amputation neuropathy (phantom limb or stump pain)
- Paraneoplastic and malignancy-related pain

Complex regional pain syndromes are likely to fall into both categories.

Sensations which may be described in neuropathic pain

- Allodynia: feeling pain in response to a usually non-painful stimulus (e.g. soft touch or temperature change)
- Hyperalgesia: exaggerated pain response to painful stimulus
- Hyperpathia: an exaggerated pain response to a repetitive stimulus

What is the management of neuropathic pain?

- Psychological techniques, e.g. cognitive behavioural therapy (CBT)
- Pharmacological management
  - Offer either amitriptyline, duloxetine, gabapentin or pregabalin initially
  - If the first option is not effective, try each of the other options or try a combination
  - Tramadol can be used in the short term as a rescue therapy
  - Capsacin cream can be used for localised pain and may be a good option for patients who cannot take oral therapies
  - Carbamazepine is first line for trigeminal neuralgia only
- Options for refractory pain
  - Percutaneous electrical nerve stimulation
  - Spinal cord stimulation
  - Specialist pain management referral

Case 13

Mrs Layupp is a 29-year-old woman who works as an employment solicitor. She has found it harder to concentrate on her cases recently, all involving difficult claims between employers and her clients. She has told her husband that she thinks it's all stress, but other symptoms have also been notable, with joint pain, some hair falling out, a 'rash' on her face and tiredness. Around 4 months ago she had been sent, but then cancelled, a first appointment in the rheumatology clinic. Another appointment was planned in the coming 3 months. In addition, she felt she had experienced episodes of wandering over the previous 2 nights and some confusion and memory problems.

This morning, she dropped her cup of tea. Hugely startled by this, she phoned her brother, who has a flexible working pattern and with whom she has a very close relationship, and she called him over to her apartment. He helped her to call in sick to her employer. They spent the morning together but she spoke some unexpected words during that time, so he decided in the end to call the GP who set up an urgent appointment that day; on assessment, the GP sent her into hospital.

On arrival at hospital, her observations were:

Respiratory rate: 14/min
Oxygen saturations: 95% on room air
Temperature: 37.4°C
Blood pressure: 159/91 mmHg
Heart rate: 80 bpm

Which categories are there in the secondary causes of hypertension in young patients?

- Endocrine causes (thyrotoxicosis, Conn's syndrome, Cushing's, phaeochromocytoma)
- Renal causes (fibromuscular hyperplasia, renal artery disease and intrinsic renal disease)
- Cardiac causes (including coarctation of the aorta)
- Rheumatological/multisystem causes (vasculitis, lupus)

TIMEPOINT  2

Around an hour after arrival, Mrs Layupp was seen initially by a resident internal medicine doctor, who was understandably concerned about the recent symptoms. A full history, examination and initial blood tests were organised. On balance, given that urgent brain imaging and rheumatological consult were clearly indicated, it was decided that she would be admitted to hospital.

Her husband had arrived soon after admission, so for the first few hours of the assessment process, both he and Mrs Layupp's brother were by her bedside.

A CT head was normal, and Mrs Layupp and her relatives were informed of this. It was planned that an MRI brain scan should be done soon.

The routine blood tests returned (Table 13.1).

The internal medicine doctor treating Mrs Layupp was asked by a medical student working with her whether she was surprised by the high

Table 13.1 Venous blood results

White cell count	3.2×10^9/L	Corrected calcium	2.26 mmol/L
Haemoglobin	112 g/L	Albumin	33 g/L
Platelets	102×10^9/L	Bilirubin	25 μmol/L
CRP	3 mg/L	Alkaline phosphatase	127 U/L
Sodium	142 mmol/L	Alanine aminotransferase	32 U/L
Potassium	5.1 mmol/L	PT	11.3 secs
Urea	3.9 mmol/L	INR	1.0
Creatinine	68 μmol/L	APTT	18 secs
Magnesium	0.77 mmol/L	APTTR	1.0
Phosphate	0.88 mmol/L	ESR	103 mm/hr

ESR but the normal CRP. She said she wasn't. The doctor treating Mrs Layupp spoke to her senior; they agreed to ensure that an ECG, chest X-ray and a range of autoantibody blood tests took place, and they arranged an urgent electronic referral to both rheumatology and neurology.

What are the common causes of thrombocytopenia (low platelets)?

- Immune mediated e.g. ITP
- Drugs e.g. alcohol, phenytoin, vancomycin, heparin
- DIC
- TTP/HUS
- Leukaemia/lymphoma
- HIV and other viruses
- Lupus
- Pancytopenia (alongside low WCC and low Hb)
- Bone marrow pathology, e.g. malignant infiltration, myelodysplastic conditions
- Dilutional, e.g. massive transfusion
- Platelet consumption – sequestration (in the spleen)

TIMEPOINT ⏱ 3

Five hours post-admission – on the acute admission ward, both Mrs Layupp's husband and brother were fully informed of the urgency of more detailed medical investigations and the upcoming specialist referrals.

The MRI scan took place and is shown below. See Figures 13.1 and 13.2.

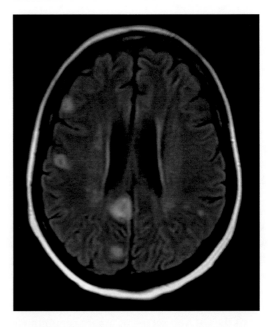

Figure 13.1 Axial fluid attenuation inversion recovery (FLAIR) MRI image through the brain.

They had some brief phone calls to make, so stepped off the ward for a short while; in that time Mrs Layupp suddenly started fitting on the ward; a number of nursing and medical team members were called to ensure positioning, airway maintenance and management of the seizure according to local protocol. Initial management included appropriately moving Mrs Layupp into the left lateral position, and the initial medication delivered was $2 \times 2 = 4$ mg lorazepam; in total, there was a 7-minute tonic clonic seizure, and given the whole overall context, the urgent calling of an anaesthetist, a rapid

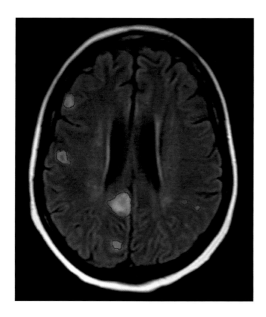

Figure 13.2 Red outline on the same FLAIR image (Figure 13.1) demonstrates numerous high signal lesions of varying sizes which are predominantly at the grey-white matter interface. Although non-specific, these appearances are highly suggestive of a cerebral vasculitis.

sequence induction and intubation took place. Several more minutes went by, and a phenytoin infusion was made up. The intensive care consultant came to the ward, arranged admission to critical care and made an immediate phone call to the duty rheumatology consultant. The phone advice to the ITU consultant from the rheumatology consultant was to add in dexamethasone 6 mg IV BD.

That same evening, all the observations had become more stable, so extubation took place, and Mrs Layupp was more settled on ITU, alert, eating and drinking. The rheumatology consultant who was phoned earlier was conscientious, pro-active and never ignored the need to see patients sooner rather than later, so went to the critical care unit around 10 pm, reviewed Mrs Layupp and concluded that she most probably had systemic lupus erythematosus with neurological involvement leading to the seizure.

The senior sister on critical care asked the rheumatologist about the factors that lead to deciding someone has lupus.

Clinical criteria for SLE

Lupus is an important multisystem disorder. It has around a 0.2% prevalence and a 9:1 female to male preponderance. Many patients have relatively mild chronic disease or occasional flares; but some patients develop severe complications including, for example, effects on the renal and nervous systems.

One parallel syndrome is known as antiphospholipid syndrome which is associated with a range of challenging thrombotic episodes and multiple miscarriages.

The SLICC clinical criteria for lupus require four or more of the features below, including at least one clinical and one laboratory feature.

CLINICAL

1. Red facial rash described as malar
2. Discoid skin changes (discoloured patches on skin with scarring)
3. Pleuritic or pericarditic inflammation – i.e. serositis
4. Ulceration (includes oral or nasopharyngeal ulcers)
5. Arthropathy: nonerosive arthritis of two or more peripheral joints, with tenderness, swelling or effusion
6. Non-scarring alopecia
7. Haemolytic anaemia
8. Low white cell count
9. Thrombocytopenia
10. Proteinuria and/or cell casts in the urine
11. Neurologic disorder: seizures or psychosis

LABORATORY

1. Positive ANA
2. Positive anti-dsDNA
3. Positive anti-Sm
4. Positive antiphospholipid antibody
5. Low complement
6. Positive direct Coombs test without haemolytic anaemia

Does SLE have a range of neurological manifestations?

Yes, they are as follows:

- Stroke
- Seizures
- Posterior reversible encephalopathy syndrome (PRES)
- Neuropsychiatric changes
- Cranial nerve alterations
- Headache
- Eye/visual changes
- Peripheral neuropathy

The rheumatologist made regular visits in the days that followed, both in critical care, then back on a regular medical ward, and was asked by Mrs Layupp's husband what, if any, treatment for the lupus was needed. The following answer was given.

Treatment of lupus

This can be categorised into mild/moderate/severe disease.

Mild disease – many mild manifestations of lupus, such as skin and joint involvement, can be treated with hydroxychloroquine and low-dose prednisone or nonsteroidal anti-inflammatory drugs.

Moderate disease – clinical manifestations, such as skin, joint, hematologic or non-life-threatening serositis, are treated with hydroxychloroquine and moderate-dose prednisone and are often also supplemented with another immunosuppressive agent, such as methotrexate, azathioprine, mycophenolate mofetil or belimumab.

Severe, organ-threatening disease – often treated with high-dose glucocorticoids and also with a glucocorticoid-sparing agent, such as cyclophosphamide, mycophenolate mofetil or azathioprine.

TIMEPOINT 4

Two months later, in the rheumatology clinic, Mrs Layupp – now significantly better – offers sincere thanks to the rheumatology consultant and specialist nurse to share with the whole medical and intensive care team as she felt she received excellent care during the very challenging recent admission. She does not remember it all, but her husband echoes a sense of such positivity. They do, however, harbour concerns about the long-term implications of her condition, both now and in the future.

Now that she has made an almost complete recovery, she asks the consultant about the question of how and when she should consider starting a family and what issues are relevant in terms of family planning and contraception in a person who has developed lupus.

What are the key considerations for preconception planning in lupus patients?

- Many women of childbearing age develop lupus
- Specialist clinics for this purpose are run in specialist centres
- Most lupus patients can have successful pregnancies
- Fetal monitoring may include Doppler ultrasonography especially in the third trimester, to screen for placental insufficiency and impaired fetal development
- Hypertensive and vaso-occlusive episodes need to be areas of vigilance

FURTHER READING

1. https://ard.bmj.com/content/76/3/476
2. https://www.ncbi.nlm.nih.gov/pmc/articles/PMC5298362/-Diagrams
3. Petri, M., Orbai, A.-M., Alarcón, G.S., et al. (2012), Derivation and validation of the Systemic Lupus International Collaborating Clinics classification criteria for systemic lupus erythematosus. *Arthritis & Rheumatism*, 64: 2677–2686. https://doi.org/10.1002/art.34473

Case 14

Mrs Jenkins is a 92-year-old woman, brought to the emergency department by her son as he has noticed that she has become jaundiced. Yesterday he thought it was a trick of the light but today he is sure that her skin and eyes appear yellow.

The emergency department doctor takes a history from Mrs Jenkins. She reports that she is feeling well and denies any abdominal or back pain. Over the last week or two she has noticed that her urine has been darker than usual, but she simply assumed that she was dehydrated and had been trying to drink more water. On direct questioning she agrees that perhaps her stools have been lighter as well. She has not noticed any weight loss. She has been a little itchy recently, but she put it down to her skin tending to become dry over the winter, and she had been using extra moisturiser to deal with this.

Her past medical history includes age-related dry macular degeneration, migraines and hypertension. The only medication she takes is amlodipine 5 mg daily, and she has no known drug allergies. She has never had any hospital admissions as all of her children were born at home. She drinks a small glass of white wine each week on a Saturday night whilst watching television, but otherwise drinks only at family occasions. She has never smoked. She is unsure of her family history as both of her parents died young. She does not really know the details as such things were not spoken about in those days and she was sent to live with her aunt.

Her observations are:

Respiratory rate: 18/min
Oxygen saturations: 95% on room air
Temperature: 36.4°C
Blood pressure: 132/84 mmHg
Heart rate: 83 bpm

Looking from the end of the bed, Mrs Jenkins has obvious scleral jaundice with jaundice visible on the skin as well. Her clothes appear slightly loose-fitting although not excessively. Cardiovascular and respiratory examinations are normal. The abdomen is soft and non-tender. There are no palpable masses, and no gross organomegaly, although the doctor is unsure if they can palpate a liver edge. Courvoisier's test is negative, and there is no Virchow's node. She has no peripheral stigmata of liver disease.

What are the aetiologies of cholestatic jaundice?

- Intrahepatic
  - Viral or alcoholic hepatitis
  - Cirrhosis of any cause
  - Primary biliary cirrhosis
  - Obstetric cholestasis
  - Drugs: contraceptive pill, steroid, erythromycin, chlorpromazine, levomepromazine, prochlorperazine, thiazide diuretics, co-amoxiclav
  - Congenital
- Extrahepatic
  - Gallstones pathologies including choledocholithiasis, ascending cholangitis and Mirizzi syndrome
  - Cholangiocarcinoma, cancer of the pancreatic head and cancer of the ampulla of Vater
  - Biliary strictures
  - Primary sclerosing cholangitis
  - Pancreatitis and pancreatic pseudocysts

The doctor is concerned about the possible implications of an elderly woman presenting with painless obstructive jaundice. An initial panel of blood tests is sent (Table 14.1).

The emergency department doctor also requests an abdominal ultrasound, which is reported as follows:

Table 14.1 Venous blood results

White cell count	13.4 × 10⁹/L	Corrected calcium	2.20 mmol/L
Haemoglobin	107 g/L	Albumin	33 g/L
Platelets	256 × 10⁹/L	Bilirubin	116 µmol/L
CRP	68 mg/L	Alkaline phosphatase	409 U/L
Sodium	137 mmol/L	Alanine aminotransferase	655 U/L
Potassium	4.2 mmol/L	PT	11.2 secs
Urea	5.1 mmol/L	INR	1.0
Creatinine	83 µmol/L	APTT	25.4 secs
Magnesium	0.83 mmol/L	APTTR	1.0
Phosphate	0.91 mmol/L	Fibrinogen	3.8 g/L

There is intrahepatic duct dilatation in the left and right lobes of the liver. No obvious solid focal liver lesions are seen. In the proximal body of the pancreas there is a solid avascular mass measuring 32 × 34 mm. The head and tail of the pancreas appear normal. No abnormality is demonstrated in the spleen or kidneys. The gallbladder contains no calculi but is overly distended. The common bile duct is dilated measuring 13 mm as it enters the liver and 18 mm in AP diameter as it enters the pancreatic head.

Mrs Jenkins is referred to the medical team and seen by a medical consultant. In light of the clinical history, deranged liver function and ultrasound results, the consultant has a high suspicion of a new diagnosis of pancreatic cancer. She therefore requests tumour markers and a staging CT scan.

Which tumour marker(s) would be most useful to send? What could cause false-positive results?

CA19-9 is the tumour marker most associated with hepatobiliary cancer. It has a sensitivity of approximately 80% and specificity of between 80 and 90% for pancreatic cancer. It has a low positive predictive value and is therefore not a useful screening tool. It also provides prognostic information in that levels are inversely correlated with survival.

False-positive CA19-9 may be caused by many hepatobiliary pathologies, including liver cirrhosis, cholestasis, cholangitis, liver abscesses and cysts, hepatitis, pancreatitis and pancreatic abscesses and pseudocysts. CA19-9 may also be raised in other hepatobiliary and gastrointestinal malignancies, diabetes and irritable bowel disease.

Her tumour markers are reported as:

Tumour marker results

CEA	4.0 ug/L
AFP	4 kU/L
CA125	12 kU/L
CA19-9	62 U/mL

Mrs Jenkins is admitted to the medical ward and referred to the hepatobiliary MDT.

A CT and MRCP are performed with select images shown below. See Figures 14.1, 14.2 and 14.3. The CT chest, abdomen and pelvis, including a dual-phase pancreatic scan, are reported as follows:

There is a 37 mm solid mass in the head of the pancreas causing marked pancreatic duct, intra- and extra-hepatic biliary ductal dilation suspicious for a neoplasm, with no definite evidence of metastasis.

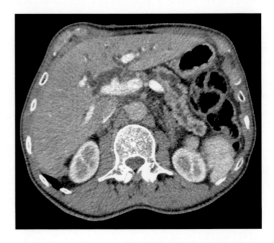

Figure 14.1 Axial, post-contrast computed tomography (CT) image through the level of the pancreas.

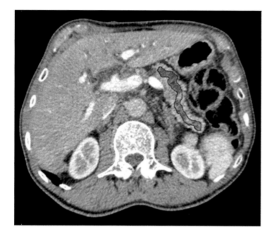

Figure 14.2 The red outline on the same image (Figure 14.1) demonstrates pancreatic duct dilatation. The blue outline indicates intra-hepatic duct dilatation.

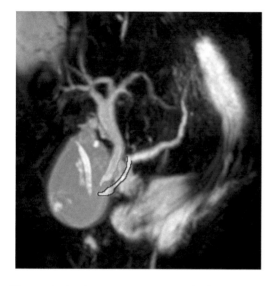

Figure 14.3 Magnetic resonance cholangio-pancreatography (MRCP) image showing the 'double duct sign'. Both the pancreatic duct (red outline) and the common bile duct (blue outline) are dilated.

Mrs Jenkins is admitted to the medical ward and referred to the hepatobiliary MDT.

TIMEPOINT ⏱ 2

Two days later, Mrs Jenkins is reviewed on the ward by the hepatobiliary clinical nurse specialist.

She tells her that the MDT have had their initial meeting, and they have agreed that they would like her to have an ERCP with biopsies in order to obtain a tissue diagnosis. She explains that no decisions have been made yet about potential treatments, and this is why the biopsies are needed. Mrs Jenkins says that she has already thought about this and discussed this with her family, and that she does not want any chemotherapy, radiotherapy or major surgery if this is what she would be offered. Mrs Jenkins is aware of the fact that her prognosis may be poor, and she would like to leave hospital as soon as possible in order to enjoy any time she has left with her children and grandchildren. The clinical nurse specialist explains that they would still like to offer her stenting during the ERCP for symptomatic relief. Mrs Jenkins agrees to this.

What are the indications for ERCP? When should MRCP be used instead, and what are the advantages and disadvantages of this imaging modality?

- Indications for ERCP
  - Sphincterotomy and stone removal
  - (Palliative) stenting of biliary obstruction
  - Dilatation of strictures
  - Tissue diagnosis of pancreatic and biliary malignancies using brushings or biopsies
- Indications for MRCP
  - Diagnosis of bile duct obstruction
  - Planning for ERCP (assessment of anatomy)
  - Pancreatic surveillance in familial syndromes
- Advantages of MRCP
  - Non-invasive
  - Comparable to ERCP for diagnosis
  - Less likely to require contrast agent
- Disadvantages of MRCP
  - Cannot be used if there are contraindications to MRI (such as metallic implants or pacemakers)
  - Unable to perform any interventions if pathology is found

- Patient may still require ERCP if the MRCP is not diagnostic

The ERCP takes place later that afternoon. Biliary brushings are sent from the common bile duct stenosis. A sphincterotomy is performed and an 8 cm metal stent is inserted which appears to be working well. Mrs Jenkins is transferred back to the ward after she recovers from the sedation.

Twelve hours later, the nurses bleep the on-call doctor as Mrs Jenkins' heart rate is 112 bpm and she is complaining of abdominal pain.

Her observations are:

Respiratory rate: 20/min
Oxygen saturations: 94% on room air
Temperature: 37.8°C
Blood pressure: 124/79 mmHg
Heart rate: 111 bpm

The on-call doctor reviews her and sends some blood tests, including an arterial blood gas (Table 14.2).

What are the common complications of ERCP?

- Pancreatitis
  - Incidence difficult to determine as definition not standardised. Very operator-dependent
  - Suggested by abdominal pain and elevated amylase and lipase on blood tests
  - Management is the same as pancreatitis from other causes
- Infection
  - Including ascending cholangitis, cholecystitis, pancreatic infection, peritonitis
- Bleeding
- Perforation of duodenum
  - Can sometimes be treated during the procedure if identified immediately
  - Otherwise may be managed conservatively or via surgical repair
- Contrast allergy
- Failure of procedure
- Anaesthetic complications

Key point

Percutaneous transhepatic cholangiography with biliary stenting and drainage is another option that may be appropriate if ERCP fails.

The on-call doctor is concerned about the possibility that Mrs Jenkins has developed pancreatitis secondary to the ERCP. He calculates her Glasgow score to determine the severity of this case.

Table 14.2 Venous and arterial blood results

White cell count	14.7×10^9/L	Amylase	1273 U/L
Haemoglobin	104 g/L	Glucose	11.8 mmol/L
Platelets	298×10^9/L	Corrected calcium	2.42 mmol/L
CRP	125 mg/L	Albumin	33 g/L
Sodium	138 mmol/L	Bilirubin	109 µmol/L
Potassium	4.5 mmol/L	ALP	387 U/L
Urea	5.9 mmol/L	ALT	498 U/L
Creatinine	92 µmol/L	LDH	345 U/L
pH	7.37		
PCO_2	5.2 kPa		
PO_2	11.3 kPa		
HCO_3	23.6 mmol/L		
Base excess	0.7 mmol/L		
Lactate	0.9 mmol/L		

What is Mrs Jenkins' Glasgow score?

Table 14.3 Glasgow score

Criterion		Present?
Age	> 55 years	✓
White cell count	> 15 × 10⁹/L	✗
Urea	> 16 mmol/L	✗
Glucose	> 10 mmol/L	✓
PO$_2$	< 8 kPa	✗
Calcium	< 2 mmol/L	✗
Albumin	< 32 g/L	✗
Lactate dehydrogenase	> 600 U/L	✗
AST or ALT	> 200 U/L	✗
	Total score =	**2**

He concludes that the pancreatitis is likely to be mild as her Glasgow score is below 3 (Table 14.3) and that Mrs Jenkins is stable for now. He makes her nil by mouth and gives her IV fluids and analgesia.

TIMEPOINT ⏱ 3

Four days after the ERCP, Mrs Jenkins is seen on the ward round (Table 14.4). She still feels quite weak and is concerned about the fact she has a headache and feels dizzy whenever she stands up.

Her observations are:

Respiratory rate: 16/min
Oxygen saturations: 96% on room air
Temperature: 36.7°C
Blood pressure: 121/83 mmHg
Heart rate: 89 bpm

The biliary brushing report is now back and notes the presence of highly atypical cells with enlarged, hyperchromatic pleomorphic nuclei suspicious of malignancy.

The drug chart is reviewed, and it is noted that she is hypoglycaemic every morning. The medical student on the team asks the consultant how they can be sure that it is not a neuroendocrine tumour.

What types of pancreatic neuroendocrine tumours are there, and what are the key distinguishing symptoms of these?

- Insulinoma
  - Fasting hypoglycaemia
  - Symptoms and signs of hypoglycaemia such as dizziness, headache, sweating, visual disturbance, confusion, amnesia, tachycardia, palpitations, anxiety, weakness, seizure
  - Whipple's triad = symptomatic hypoglycaemia + plasma glucose ≤2.2 mmol/L + resolution of symptoms with glucose
- Gastrinoma
  - Abdominal pain
  - Peptic ulceration refractory to medications (Zollinger–Ellison syndrome)
  - Reflux and dysphagia
  - Diarrhoea and steatorrhoea
- Glucagonoma
  - Skin, hair and nails: necrolytic migratory erythema, alopecia and onycholysis
  - Mucous membranes: urethritis, vulvovaginitis, angular stomatitis

Table 14.4 Venous blood results

White cell count	14.2 × 10⁹/L	Amylase	103 U/L
Haemoglobin	109 g/L	Glucose	3.2 mmol/L
Platelets	314 × 10⁹/L	Corrected calcium	2.36 mmol/L
CRP	72 mg/L	Albumin	34 g/L
Sodium	136 mmol/L	Bilirubin	73 µmol/L
Potassium	3.9 mmol/L	ALP	247 U/L
Urea	5.2 mmol/L	ALT	183 U/L
Creatinine	78 µmol/L	LDH	214 U/L

- Metabolic: glucose intolerance which may ultimately lead to diabetes mellitus, weight loss
  - Psychiatric: depression, psychosis
- VIPoma (vasoactive intestinal polypeptide secreting tumours)
  - Severe watery diarrhoea leading to abdominal pain, weakness, hypotension, weight loss and hypokalaemia
  - Achlorhydria
- Somatostatinoma
  - Diabetes mellitus
  - Anaemia
  - Cholelithiasis
  - Diarrhoea, steatorrhoea and weight loss
- Carcinoid tumours
  - Flushing (especially facial)
  - Tachycardia and palpitations
  - Breathlessness and wheeze
  - Diarrhoea, abdominal pain and anorexia

Insulinomas are the most common functional pancreatic neuroendocrine tumours. How might Mrs Jenkins be investigated for an insulinoma and managed, in the context of a known pancreatic mass?

- Investigation
  - Evidence of fasting hypoglycaemia (72-hour fast is gold standard)
  - Elevated proinsulin, C-peptide and insulin levels
  - Low β-hydroxybutyrate level
  - Imaging such as US for localisation, and CT or MRI for staging already done
- Management
  - Pharmacological
    - Management of electrolyte abnormalities, e.g. potassium and glucose replacement
    - Management of hypoglycaemia with diazoxide and somatostatin analogues such as octreotide
    - Chemotherapy
    - Other drugs rarely used such as interferon and everolimus

- Surgery
  - Resectable via (partial) pancreatectomy or Whipple procedure in the majority
  - May also use debulking surgery for palliation

TIMEPOINT 4

Four weeks later, Mrs Jenkins is seen in hepatobiliary clinic with her eldest son. He asks if it would be possible for him to have genetic testing for pancreatic cancer. He is concerned about the possibility of a familial cancer syndrome as he has read that up to 15% of pancreatic cancers are genetic.

How would you approach his concerns in terms of history taking?

- The patient should be asked about their medical history in detail
- Questions should also be asked about the patient's children and partner (and any previous partners), followed by questions about the patient's parents, siblings and their partners, nieces, nephews, grandparents, aunts, uncles and first cousins (i.e. to include all first- and second-degree relatives over three generations). It may be necessary to do the same with the patient's partner
- It is generally useful to draw a family pedigree tree. An excellent explanation for how these should be drawn is available on the NHS National Genetics and Genomics Education Centre website: www.genomicseducation.hee.nhs.uk/takingfamilyhistory101/how-do-i-draw-a-family-history/
- The following information should be included
  - Date of birth and birth defects
  - Ethnic background
  - Date of death and cause
  - Major medical problems and age of onset
  - Major risk factors, e.g. smoking status, weight
  - Pregnancies and their outcomes including unborn children, miscarriages, stillbirths and neonatal deaths

In this situation, if evidence of a possible family history were uncovered, it might be appropriate to discuss testing for BRCA1, BRCA2, PRSS1 and PALB2 with a geneticist as all of these are associated with an increased risk of pancreatic cancer.

Which familial syndromes should be considered in patients with pancreatic tumours and a possible family history?

- Peutz–Jeghers syndrome
  - Autosomal dominant disorder caused by mutation in STK11 tumour suppressor gene
  - Associated with hamartomatous polyps of the gastrointestinal tract, melanosis (hyperpigmented macules on the oral mucosa, hands and feet) and an increased risk of many cancers including pancreatic
- Familial atypical multiple mole and melanoma syndrome
  - Caused by faults in CDKN2A and CDK4 genes
  - Associated with multiple naevi, cutaneous and ocular malignant melanomas, as well as pancreatic cancer
- Lynch syndrome (hereditary non-polyposis colorectal cancer)
  - Autosomal dominant disorder caused by mutations in MLH1, MSH2, MSH6 or PMS2 genes
  - Extremely high lifetime risk of colorectal cancer, but also high risk for hepatobiliary, endometrial, ovarian and gastric cancers
- Von Hippel–Lindau syndrome
  - Autosomal dominant disorder caused by mutation in VHL tumour suppressor gene
  - Leads to haemangiomas developing in the central nervous system and retina
  - Also strongly associated with phaeochromocytomas, endolymphatic sac tumours, renal and pancreatic cysts, clear cell renal cell carcinoma and pancreatic neuroendocrine tumours
- Multiple endocrine neoplasia type 1
  - Autosomal dominant disorder caused by a mutation in the MEN1 tumour suppressor gene
  - Causes parathyroid hyperplasia/adenoma, pancreatic neuroendocrine tumours and pituitary adenomas
- Familial adenomatous polyposis or Gardner's syndrome
  - Caused by APC gene if inherited in autosomal dominant pattern, or MUTYH gene if inherited in an autosomal recessive pattern
  - Associated with large numbers of colonic polyps which have a tendency to undergo malignant transformation. Patients may also have osteomas, epidermal cysts, dermoid tumours and fibromas. It is also associated with an increased risk of gastric and hepatobiliary cancers
- Li–Fraumeni syndrome
  - Autosomal dominant syndrome caused by mutations in the TP53 tumour suppressor gene or the CHEK2 tumour suppressor gene
  - Associated with increased risk of breast cancer, osteosarcomas, soft tissue sarcomas, brain tumours, leukaemia and pancreatic cancer

Case 15

Mr Blake is a 23-year-old student nurse who attends his GP as he is concerned about a red, blotchy, painful rash on his shins. He is very upset about the cosmetic appearance of this rash as he swims regularly and feels everyone at the pool is staring at his legs. He reports that he has felt generally fatigued lately, and also mentions that he has been a little worried about having diarrhoea with some intermittent abdominal pain over the last few weeks. However, he had put his symptoms down to a mixture of poor diet and stress and had assumed they would improve by themselves. He thinks that the diarrhoea can now occur up to five times a day, and sometimes has blood in it, but not always. He thinks he has probably lost some weight as a result but hadn't been worried as he had been keen to lose a few pounds anyway. He is still eating and drinking normally and has not had any change to his appetite. All of his symptoms have started within the last 6 weeks.

He has no significant past medical or surgical history. No-one in his family has anything similar that he is aware of. He has not travelled abroad recently. He drinks 8–10 units of alcohol a week, and smokes 15 cigarettes a day. On examination he appears generally well, if a little pale.

His observations are:

Respiratory rate: 16/min
Oxygen saturations: 100% on room air
Temperature: 36.2°C
Blood pressure: 105/76 mmHg
Heart rate: 79 bpm

He has conjunctival pallor, and his mucous membranes appear dry. Otherwise, his cardiovascular and respiratory examinations are normal. His abdomen is soft and mildly tender, although he struggles to pinpoint the location of the pain. There is no organomegaly and no other masses are palpable. On examination of the lower legs, the rash appears symmetrical bilaterally and consists of multiple erythematous nodules approximately 2–3 cm in diameter. The lesions are very tender to palpation.

What initial investigations would it be appropriate to do to investigate for inflammatory bowel disease, and why?

- Full blood count: anaemia secondary to malabsorption
- Urea and electrolytes, including magnesium and calcium levels: dehydration and electrolyte abnormalities secondary to diarrhoea and malabsorption
- Liver function tests, including albumin: malabsorption
- ESR: evidence of an inflammatory process
- Ferritin, B12 and folate: abnormalities secondary to malabsorption
- Tissue transglutaminase (TTG): Coeliac disease
- Fecal calprotectin: inflammatory bowel disease
- Stool cultures: evidence of *Clostridium difficile* or *Escherichia coli* 0157:H7

Serology testing

Serology testing may be useful in secondary care:

- Positive anti-*Saccharomyces cerevisiae* antibodies (ASCA) alone have a high positive predictive value and specificity for Crohn's disease
- Positive perinuclear antineutrophil cytoplasmic antibodies (p-ANCA) with a negative ASCA are very specific for ulcerative colitis patients in IBD cohorts

DOI: 10.1201/9781351257725-15

The GP explains that he thinks the rash may be linked to the diarrhoea, and he is concerned about a possible diagnosis of inflammatory bowel disease. He tells Mr Blake that he would like to do some initial tests as well as an urgent gastroenterology referral.

Before he leaves the surgery, Mr Blake provides blood and stool samples. The GP reviews the results later that evening before writing a referral letter (Table 15.1).

The GP phones Mr Blake and asks him to collect a prescription for 20 mg prednisolone. He asks him to take one tablet daily until he sees the gastroenterologist as he strongly suspects inflammatory bowel disease and is keen to induce remission as soon as possible. He understands the plan and agrees to do this.

What are the other extra-intestinal manifestations of IBD?

- Rheumatological — Arthritis, ankylosing spondylitis, sacroiliitis
- Bone — Osteoporosis, osteopenia, osteonecrosis
- Ophthalmological — Uveitis, episcleritis, iritis, conjunctivitis
- Skin — Erythema nodosum, pyoderma gangrenosum
- Hepatological — Primary sclerosing cholangitis, autoimmune liver disease
- Miscellaneous — Aphthous ulcers, clubbing

TIMEPOINT 🕐 2

Mr Blake is reviewed in the gastroenterology clinic 4 weeks later. Due to having a positive fecal calprotectin, he was offered a rapid access endoscopy prior to his clinic appointment. His endoscopy report is as follows:

Procedure performed
Colonoscopy – complete to terminal ileum.

Indications for examination
Increasing frequency of diarrhoea, with intermittent blood in stool.

Procedure
Informed consent was obtained, patient prepped in left lateral position. Once conscious sedation was achieved the colonoscope was introduced into the rectum and advanced under direct visualisation to the terminal ileum. Adequate bowel prep. The scope was subsequently withdrawn with five biopsies taken at separate sites. The procedure was tolerated well and uncomplicated, and Mr Blake was transferred to the recovery bay with no concerns.

Findings
Focal ulceration adjacent to normal mucosa, leading to a cobblestone appearance with skip lesions. Multiple granulomata demonstrated.

Endoscopic diagnosis
Crohn's disease.

Table 15.1 Venous blood results

White cell count	9.6×10^9/L	Corrected calcium	2.25 mmol/L
Haemoglobin	103 g/L	Magnesium	0.71 mmol/L
Platelets	392×10^9/L	Albumin	31 g/L
MCV	71 fL	Bilirubin	6 µmol/L
ESR	6 mm/hr	Alkaline phosphatase	42 U/L
Sodium	138 mmol/L	Alanine aminotransferase	21 U/L
Potassium	3.3 mmol/L	B12	202 g/L
Urea	5.6 mmol/L	Folate	5.2 ng/mL
Creatinine	97 µmol/L	Ferritin	31 µg/L
Tissue transglutaminase (TTG)	8 U/mL (negative)		

Recommendations

For urgent gastroenterology review. Await biopsy results.

Mr Blake tells the gastroenterology consultant that he feels his symptoms are getting worse despite the prednisolone.

How is disease severity classified in inflammatory bowel disease?

One way in which Crohn's disease severity can be calculated is using the Crohn's Disease Activity Index (CDAI). This is the gold standard; however, it is a very complex calculation, best done using a calculator where the values can be inputted. It takes into account the number of soft stools, abdominal pain ratings, general wellbeing, signs of extra-intestinal disease and weight loss, amongst other things. Having a CDAI of between 150 and 1100 suggests active Crohn's disease. A higher score suggests more severe disease activity.

For ulcerative colitis, NICE recommends the Truelove and Witt's severity index (Table 15.2).

As Mr Blake now has a CDAI of 290, the gastroenterologist says that he would like to add in another drug called azathioprine.

Did you know?

Patients should be tested for TPMT levels prior to starting on azathioprine or other thioprine-based drugs. Patients deficient in the TPMT enzyme which metabolises thioprine drugs may experience severe and potentially dangerous side effects if they are given therapeutic doses.

What are key medications and classes of medication used in IBD?

Table 15.3 covers the key classes of medications used in inflammatory bowel disease.

There are other medications which may be used by specialists, such as:

- Immunosuppressant drugs, e.g. tacrolimus and ciclosporin are both used for UC
- Monoclonal antibodies
    - Anti-TNF agents, e.g. infliximab and adalimumab may be used to induce remission in severe CD that has not responded to other treatments. It is rarely needed as maintenance treatment
    - Vedolizumab is an integrin $\alpha 4 \beta 7$ monoclonal antibody used in the treatment of severe CD and UC

TIMEPOINT 🕐 3

Four months later, Mr Blake is brought to the emergency department by ambulance. The paramedics explain in their handover that they think he is very dehydrated, so have already cannulated him and started fluids on the way to the hospital. The doctor agrees so he has another cannula inserted and bloods taken by the staff nurse and sent urgently while he talks to the doctor. He reports that over the last 5 days he has lost count of the number of episodes of bloody diarrhoea that he has had. He thought that it would pass by itself, but as it is still ongoing he was planning to visit his GP tomorrow. However, since this morning he has started to feel unwell in himself,

Table 15.2 Truelove and Witt's severity index

	Mild	Moderate	Severe
Number of stools/day	<4	4–6	>6
Blood in stools	Very small	Small	Clearly visible
Severe disease should include at least one of the following features:			
Anaemia	None	None	Anaemia
Pulse	<90	<90	>90
Fever	None	None	Above 37.8°C
ESR	Normal	Normal	>30

Table 15.3 Key medications used in inflammatory bowel disease

Medication	Usage				Side effects	Monitoring
	CD: Induce remission	CD: Maintain remission	UC: Induce remission	UC: Maintain remission		
Steroids, e.g. prednisolone, methylprednisolone, IV hydrocortisone, budesonide	✓	✗	✓	✓	GI side effects, insomnia, mood change, hyperglycaemia	None required for short-term courses, but blood glucose should be checked in diabetic patients
Aminosalicylate(5-ASA) drugs, e.g. sulfasalazine, mesalazine	✓	✗	✓	✗	GI side effects, headache, myalgia, arthralgia, yellow/orange discolouration of urine/contact lenses with sulfasalazine	Should not be taken by patients with G6PD deficiency or porphyria Requires monitoring for agranulocytosis
TMPT drugs, e.g. azathioprine, mercaptopurine	✓	✓	✗	✓	Nausea, anorexia	TMPT levels should be checked before starting Monitor for agranulocytosis: FBC weekly for 4 weeks, then 3-monthly
Methotrexate	✓	✓	✗	✗	GI side effects, headache, fever	Contraception required during treatment and for 3 months after (men and women) Risk of agranulocytosis, renal and hepatic problems: check FBC, U&E and LFT every 1–2 weeks until on stable dose, and then every 2–3 months Folic acid should be given on days when methotrexate is not being taken

and his girlfriend says that she has brought him in today because he 'just looks awful', and called the ambulance because he was so weak and exhausted that he could barely stand. In particular she has noticed that his stomach has started to puff up weirdly which is really worrying her. Mr Blake says that his abdominal pain is getting worse and worse but denies any other specific symptoms.

Upon observation from the end of the bed, Mr Blake appears unwell. His observations are:

Respiratory rate: 26/min
Oxygen saturations: 98% on room air
Temperature: 38.9°C
Blood pressure: 92/70 mmHg
Heart rate: 126 bpm

On examination, he is cool peripherally with a capillary refill time of 3 seconds. His heart sounds and breathing sounds are normal although he is very tachycardic and tachypnoeic. The abdomen is tender with guarding and rebound tenderness in all quadrants, and significantly distended.

The doctor reviews Mr Blake's initial blood results which are starting to come back (Table 15.4). He is aware of Mr Blake's history of inflammatory bowel disease and is concerned about the possibility of a toxic megacolon.

He requests an urgent abdominal X-ray. See Figure 15.1.

What are the criteria for diagnosis of toxic megacolon?

The most commonly used are the Jalan criteria, which are:

- Radiographic evidence of acute colitis, i.e. ≥6 cm colonic dilatation on abdominal X-ray

PLUS three out of four of:

- Fever > 38.6°C
- Heart rate > 120 bpm
- White cell count > 10.5 × 10⁹/L
- Anaemia

PLUS one of:

Table 15.4 Venous blood results

White cell count	18.3 × 10⁹/L
Haemoglobin	99 g/L
Platelets	413 × 10⁹/L
MCV	72 fL
CRP	298 mg/L
Sodium	135 mmol/L
Potassium	2.9 mmol/L
Urea	8.7 mmol/L
Creatinine	115 µmol/L

- Evidence of dehydration
- Altered mental status
- Electrolyte abnormalities
- Hypotension

The resus doctor reviews the Jalan criteria and thinks that this qualifies as a case of toxic megacolon. He bleeps the surgical registrar to ask them to review Mr Blake urgently, and asks what he can do until they arrive.

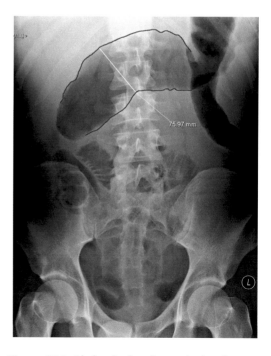

Figure 15.1 Abdominal radiograph showing a featureless, dilated transverse colon (outlined in red).

What is the management of toxic megacolon?

- Investigations
  - Blood tests to include: full blood count, urea and electrolytes, liver function tests, coagulation screen, group and save, blood cultures
  - Stool cultures
  - Abdominal X-ray and erect chest X-ray
- IV fluid resuscitation
- Catheter to permit strict input/output monitoring
- Complete bowel rest – patient should be made nil by mouth
- Insertion of a nasogastric tube for decompression of the bowel
- Stop aminosalicylate drugs, opiates, anti-motility agents and anticholingeric agents
- Give broad-spectrum antibiotics and intravenous steroid

Mr Blake is reviewed by the surgical registrar who agrees to take over his care. He is managed conservatively on the surgical ward. Unfortunately, after 48 hours there has been no improvement in his condition, so he undergoes a subtotal colectomy with formation of an end ileostomy. He makes a good recovery from the operation, and his medications are optimised again. Ten days later, Mr Blake is discharged back to the care of gastroenterology in the community, with additional support from the community stoma nurses.

TIMEPOINT ⏱ 4

Three years later, Mr Blake presents to the emergency department as he is unable to tolerate any oral intake. Over the last 5 days he has been vomiting numerous times each day. He thinks that he has caught a vomiting bug from his 18-month-old daughter as there are always lots of infections going around her nursery and she has also been unwell over the last few days. He is feeling very fatigued and has a bad headache. Over the last couple of months he has also had increasingly loose stoma output which he is now finding difficult to manage. He has noticed when he

is changing the bags that the content has become extremely smelly. He thinks that recently he has lost some weight without intending to, but still thinks he looks the same because he is bloated. Since his subtotal colectomy 3 years ago, Mr Blake has undergone two further operations to resect parts of his ileum due to stricturing from the Crohn's disease.

His observations are:

Respiratory rate: 22/min
Oxygen saturations: 97% on room air
Temperature: 37.6°C
Blood pressure: 101/75 mmHg
Heart rate: 98 bpm

On examination, he appears tired and pale. He has multiple aphthous ulcers but his general examination is otherwise normal. He appears to be underweight, and his BMI is calculated as 16.9. His initial blood results are shown in Table 15.5.

What is the best explanation for his current clinical picture?

There is evidence of malabsorption in Mr Blake's blood results, as suggested by low levels of all electrolytes. This is likely to be secondary to short bowel syndrome. Short bowel syndrome occurs in patients who have had large amounts of bowel surgically resected or damaged. As a result, these patients have a reduced capacity to absorb nutrients from their diet. This is also suggested by the history of increasingly loose and offensive-smelling stool. Symptoms and severity are variable and do not seem to correlate well with the amount of bowel resected, due to the ability of the bowel to compensate.

The emergency doctor agrees that it is likely that he has caught a vomiting bug acutely, but she is also concerned about the longer history suggestive of malabsorption.

She explains to Mr Blake that she would like to give him fluids and that his electrolytes need to be replaced appropriately in order that he doesn't become more unwell. She also explains that she would like to get an opinion from a dietician about the best long-term strategy for his diet. The emergency department doctor calls the dietician who

Table 15.5 Venous blood results

White cell count	7.4×10^9/L	Creatinine	89 µmol/L
Haemoglobin	89 g/L	Corrected calcium	1.95 mmol/L
Platelets	275×10^9/L	Magnesium	0.58 mmol/L
MCV	74 fL	Albumin	28 g/L
CRP	62 mg/L	Chloride	87 mmol/L
Sodium	142 mmol/L	B12	184 ng/L
Potassium	3.1 mmol/L	Phosphate	0.57 mmol/L
Urea	4.7 mmol/L		

agrees to come and review Mr Blake later in the afternoon, but advises that the doctor should be careful as Mr Blake is at high risk of refeeding syndrome.

What are the risk factors for refeeding syndrome?

Refeeding syndrome is when potentially dangerous shifts occur in the levels of fluids and electrolytes in patients when feeding is restarted after malabsorption or starvation. It is most common in patients receiving some form of artificial feed, but it can also occur with oral feeding, particularly if the patient is receiving nutritional supplements. The risk is increased with any cause of malabsorption.

According to the NICE guidelines, the patient is at high risk if they have:

ONE or more of the following:

- Minimal/no nutritional intake for >10 days
- Hypokalaemia, hypophosphataemia or hypomagnesaemia prior to commencing feeding
- BMI <16
- Unintentional weight loss >15% over 3–6 months

Or TWO or more of the following:

- Minimal/no nutritional intake for >5 days
- BMI <18.5

- Unintentional weight loss >10% over 3–6 months
- History of alcohol misuse or if the patient is using insulin, chemotherapy, antacids or diuretics

How can refeeding syndrome be avoided in high-risk patients?

- Appropriate dietician input
- Cautious introduction of calories, gradually titrated up
- Cardiac monitoring should be considered in extremely high-risk patients or patients with pre-existing heart conditions
- Fluid balance must be carefully monitored
- Give the following oral supplements for the first 10 days
  - Thiamine (200–300 mg OD)
  - Vitamin B co-strong (1–2 tablets TDS)
  - A balanced multivitamin (OD)
- Give the following supplementation unless levels are already high (it is **not** necessary to correct low levels prior to starting feeding)
  - Potassium (usual requirement 2–4 mmol/kg/day)
  - Phosphate (usual requirement 0.3–0.6 mmol/kg/day)
  - Magnesium (usual requirement 0.2 mmol/kg/day)

Case 16

TIMEPOINT 1

Mr Southern is a 32-year-old man who presents to the emergency department with abdominal pain. He had been playing in a football match earlier that day when he was hit by the ball on his back. His abdominal pain became progressively worse, and then he saw blood in his urine when he went to the toilet, so his girlfriend persuaded him to attend ED. Mr Southern describes that he was passing frank red blood, rather than blood-tinged urine.

He has no past medical history of note and takes no regular medications. He denies having any significant family history. He smokes around 5 cigarettes a day and drinks around 15 units of alcohol a week. He works in marketing and lives with his girlfriend and their two daughters.

His observations are:

Respiratory rate: 18/min
Oxygen saturations: 99% on room air
Temperature: 37.5°C
Blood pressure: 160/90 mmHg
Heart rate: 106 bpm

On examination, there is a palpable right flank fullness and tenderness with no associated bruising, abdominal guarding or rigidity. There is no hepatosplenomegaly. Bowel sounds are present. Systems examination is otherwise normal.

How can a kidney be differentiated from a liver or spleen on examination?

See Table 16.1.

What is the differential diagnosis for renal enlargement on palpation?

See Table 16.2.

A urine sample reveals macroscopic haematuria with urine dipstick only positive to blood (3+).
Bloods show the following:

Venous blood results

White cell count	10×10^9/L
CRP	10 mg/L
Haemoglobin	145 g/L
Platelets	225×10^9/L
Urea	10.2 mmol/L
Creatinine	192 µmol/L

He has no previous blood tests on the computer system available for comparison.

The emergency department doctor starts IV fluids, given Mr Southern's tachycardia, haematuria and probable kidney injury. He also sends off a coagulation screen and group and save samples. After this, he inserts a three-way catheter for irrigation and requests an ultrasound KUB.

The USKUB report is available later that afternoon. It shows multiple cysts in both kidneys. The emergency department doctor discusses the case with his consultant who suggests that it may be autosomal dominant polycystic kidney disease (ADPKD).

What is ADPKD?

- ADPKD is the most common inherited serious renal disorder in adults. It occurs in

DOI: 10.1201/9781351257725-16

Table 16.1 Differentiating liver and spleen on examination

	Renal mass	Liver or spleen
Palpable above	✓	X
Ballotable	✓	X
Movement with respiration	(✓)	✓
Percussion note	Resonant	Dull

Table 16.2 Differential diagnosis for renal enlargement

Unilateral	Bilateral
Polycystic kidney (with one palpable kidney)	Polycystic kidneys
Hydronephrosis	Bilateral hydronephrosis
Renal tumour	Bilateral renal tumours (e.g. renal cell carcinoma in von Hippel–Lindau syndrome)
Hypertrophy of a single working kidney	Infiltrative disease (e.g. amyloidosis)

approximately 1 in every 400 to 1000 live births
- It is inherited in an autosomal dominant fashion with two subtypes
  - ADPKD1 (~90% of cases) with the PKD1 gene located on chromosome 16
  - ADPKD2 with the PKD2 gene located on chromosome 4. It tends to have a milder phenotype with cysts occurring later on in life
  - The disease may also occasionally arise from a spontaneous mutation
- The hallmark of the disease is the continuous development of renal cysts, leading to an increase in total kidney volume and progressive renal failure

- More than 50% of patients over the age of 60 years will be dialysis-dependent, and ADPKD accounts for about 10% of all end-stage renal failure (ESRF) cases in the UK

Diagnostic criteria for ADPKD

- Important factors in establishing a diagnosis of ADPKD are the presence of a family history, the number and type of renal cysts and the age of the patient
- In a patient with no known family history, there are no specific ultrasound criteria, but there should be a high suspicion if there are more than ten cysts in each kidney
- (NB: incidental renal cysts are found on ultrasound in around 2% if under 50 years, 10–50% if over 50 years)
- Positive family history – exact criteria depend on the familial genotype
- For example, in patients with a family history of type 1 ADPKD
  - Age <30 years: at least two unilateral/bilateral renal cysts
  - Age 30–59 years: at least two cysts in each kidney
  - Age >60 years: at least four cysts in each kidney
  - The diagnosis is supported by presence of pancreatic or hepatic cysts
- Genetic testing may be required to clarify the diagnosis

Mr Southern goes on to have a CT angiogram which confirms haemorrhage into a cyst. His pain and bleeding are managed conservatively and settle after 2 days. He is discharged home with outpatient follow-up in the renal clinic.

TIMEPOINT ⏱ 2

Three months later, Mr Southern attends his first appointment in the renal clinic. He has been well since his hospital admission, but the diagnosis has come as quite a shock, and he is concerned about the implications it may have for his future, and that of his two daughters (aged 4 and 6 years). Mr Southern says that he has done some reading about the problems he may have with his kidneys.

What are some of the renal manifestations of ADPKD?

It can present with a range of symptoms, including:

- Haematuria due to rupture of a cyst into the collecting duct system
- Mild concentrating defect leading to increased thirst, polyuria, nocturia and frequency
- Nephrolithiasis
- Flank and abdominal pain
  - Acute: nephrolithiasis, infection, cyst haemorrhage
  - Chronic: capsular stretching or traction on renal pedicle
- Development of ESRF and eventual need for renal replacement therapy

Mr Southern asks if it is possible to have any problems outside of his kidneys.

What are some of the extra-renal manifestations of ADPKD?

- Polycythaemia (due to excess erythropoietin production)
- Hypertension (due to excess renin production)
- Cardiac valve disease, most commonly mitral valve prolapse and aortic regurgitation, less frequently mitral and/or tricuspid regurgitation

- Cysts in other organs, most commonly the liver, pancreas, spleen
- Cerebral aneurysms with the risk of potential subarachnoid or intracerebral haemorrhage
- Colonic diverticula
- Abdominal wall and inguinal hernias
- Rarely: male infertility due to cysts in seminal vesicles, pancreatitis due to pancreatic cysts

The risk of renal cell cancer does not appear to be higher amongst patients with ADPKD.

He also asks whether his daughters could be screened for ADPKD.

What advice should be given regarding ADPKD screening?

Some individuals may want to be screened for ADPKD. Benefits might include:

- Early detection
- Family planning
- Planning for potential organ transplantation

Screening is not advised in asymptomatic children because:

- There is a high rate of false negative results of ultrasound screening in children, since the absence of cysts does not rule out a diagnosis
- It can be argued that the consequences of a positive diagnosis (for example the emotional impact, and potential impact on the patient's education, employment and insurance issues) would outweigh the potential benefits, especially since effective therapies are not available
- It may be more appropriate to screen children for hypertension as this is a treatable complication

TIMEPOINT ⏱ 3

Six weeks later, Mr Southern presents to his GP feeling generally unwell with nausea, right flank tenderness and a temperature of 38.2°C. A urine dipstick is negative for blood, nitrites and leucocytes.

Does a negative urine dipstick rule out an infection?

- The urine dipstick may be negative in the case of a cyst infection, as the cyst may not be in direct communication with the collecting system
- Cyst infections are most commonly caused by a Gram-negative enteric organism, with *E. coli* accounting for about 75% of cases
- When deciding on antibiotic therapy, it is important to choose a lipid-soluble drug that can enter the cyst through diffusion rather than relying on a mechanism such as glomerular filtration. These include ciprofloxacin and levofloxacin, co-trimoxazole and chloramphenicol
- It is sometimes difficult to differentiate a cyst infection from pyelonephritis, although the latter tends to have a positive urine dipstick and the presence of white cell casts in the urine sediment. In addition nephrolithiasis (including staghorn calculi) may be a source of UTI in ADPKD, usually identified by imaging

When should urine dipsticks not be used for the diagnosis of a urinary tract infection?

- Urine dipsticks are not reliable in patients over 65 years
- Over 50% of non-catheterised adults over 65 will have asymptomatic bacteriuria
- This does not indicate an infection and antibiotics should not be started on the basis of a urine dip alone
- A positive urine dip should be treated if
  - The patient is symptomatic (dysuria, new urinary frequency, new urinary urgency, new incontinence, abdominal/flank pain, nausea/vomiting, fevers/rigors, new delirium, visible haematuria)
  - A urine culture is positive

The GP calls up the medical registrar of the local hospital and explains her concerns about a possible cyst infection. The medical registrar agrees to admit Mr Southern for a course of IV antibiotics. Mr Southern makes a good recovery and is discharged home 7 days later.

TIMEPOINT 4

Two years after his diagnosis, Mr Southern attends for his annual follow-up in the renal clinic. Over the past year, he has been suffering from recurrent urinary tract infections, which have often been complicated by multi-drug resistance. As a result, he has required six hospital admissions over the last year for intravenous antibiotics. The renal consultant explains that his case has been discussed in the renal MDT, and they would like to offer Mr Southern a right-sided nephrectomy, as most of his infections have originated from that side.

What are the indications for nephrectomy in ADPKD?

- Recurrent infection
- Renal haemorrhage where intra-arterial embolisation is either unsuccessful or contraindicated
- Malignancy
- To provide space for renal transplant into potential pelvic surgical site
- Limitation of daily activities due to fatigue, anorexia and pain
- Development of ventral hernia due to renomegaly

The renal consultant warns that depending on the function of the left kidney, this may predicate the need for renal replacement therapy (RRT) in the near future. He gives Mr Southern a leaflet with the various options available.

When should RRT be considered?

RRT includes:

- Haemodialysis (home- or hospital-based)
- Peritoneal dialysis
- Transplantation (cadaveric or living donor)

The indications for RRT are as follows:

- CKD
  - Patients typically begin dialysis when GFR falls below 10–15 mL/min
  - Ideally, any patient with obviously deteriorating renal function should be assessed at an early stage
- AKI
  - Pulmonary oedema not responsive to diuretics
  - Hyperkalaemia >6.5 mmol/L refractory to medical treatment
  - Severe hypernatraemia (Na >155 mmol/L) or hyponatraemia (Na <120 mmol/L)
  - Acidosis (pH <7) not responding to sodium bicarbonate
  - Uraemia
  - Drug toxicity (if drug is renally excreted)
  - Severe AKI (urea >30 mmol/L and creatinine >500 µmol/L)

RRT may not be appropriate in all patients, especially frail patients or those with multiple comorbidities. Conservative management may include dietary adaptations, symptomatic management (e.g. anti-emetics) and treatments which replace kidney functions such as erythropoietin.

Case 17

Mrs North is a 57-year-old woman who presents to the emergency department with a 2-week history of increasing shortness of breath and chest pain. She reports that her chest pain is worse on deep inspiration, and she has had a dry cough as well. She denies coughing up any blood. She has had no recent weight loss or change in appetite. She has a history of COPD, a right-sided frozen shoulder and depression. Her only regular medication is sertraline 50 mg OD, an umeclidinium/vilanterol inhaler OD and a salbutamol inhaler which she uses as required. She has a 40 pack-year history but has never drunk alcohol as she 'doesn't like the taste'. She lives alone and does not have any immediate family. She worked for 40 years as a painter and decorator, but has been unable to work for the last 2 weeks because of her breathing difficulties. She last travelled 6 weeks ago when she went on a cruise around the Mediterranean.

Her observations are:

Respiratory rate: 22/min
Oxygen saturations: 92% on room air
Temperature: 37.7°C
Blood pressure: 140/80 mmHg
Heart rate: 105 bpm

On examination, clubbing of the nails is noted. Heart sounds are normal, and Mrs North is warm and well perfused peripherally. On examination of the chest, there is reduced air entry at the left base with some fine crepitations in the left mid-zone. Systems examination is otherwise normal. A urine dip is negative.

Bloods show the following:

Venous blood results

White cell count	18.7×10^9/L
CRP	302 mg/L
Haemoglobin	102 g/L
MCV	87 fL
Platelets	457×10^9/L
Sodium	141 mmol/L
Potassium	4.6 mmol/L
Urea	5.7 mmol/L
Creatinine	87 µmol/L

Liver function and coagulation tests are normal.

Given the recent travel history and the blood tests, the emergency department doctor is concerned that Mrs North might have an atypical pneumonia. Unfortunately, Mrs North has still not had her chest X-ray, but the emergency department doctor starts treatment anyway.

Which are the most common organisms causing atypical pneumonias?

- Mycoplasma pneumoniae
- Chlamydia pneumoniae
- Legionella pneumophila

Mrs North finally goes for her chest X-ray, shown below. See Figures 17.1 and 17.2.

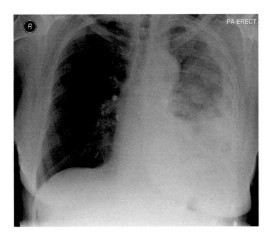

Figure 17.1 Posteroanterior (PA) chest X-ray for Mrs North.

The emergency department doctor is worried about the chest X-ray appearance so she refers Mrs North to the respiratory team for ongoing management.

What does the X-ray show, and what is the significance of this?

Pleural plaques occur in up to 60% of people exposed to asbestos and are usually

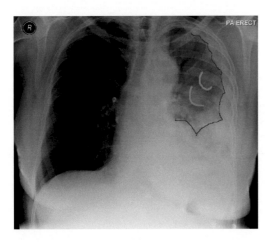

Figure 17.2 PA chest X-ray showing pleural thickening in the left hemithorax (red outline). The blue outline indicates the presence of further abnormal soft tissue. Masses which 'fade out' are likely to originate from the pleura.

asymptomatic. They are benign and do not affect lung function but may be an independent risk factor for mesothelioma. Pleural thickening may also occur after asbestos exposure although there are many other causes. Severe pleural thickening may cause shortness of breath and a restrictive defect on spirometry.

TIMEPOINT 2

The next day, Mrs North is seen by the consultant on the respiratory ward. He is concerned about the appearance of the chest X-ray, so he asks the junior doctor to arrange an urgent CT chest, abdomen and pelvis, and to take an occupational history after the ward round.

What should the junior doctor ask in an occupational history?

- Include current and previous jobs and dates
- Full time/part time/shift work?
- Job title is not enough – ask about the specific types of tasks the patient does day to day
- Specific occupational exposures
  - Chemicals/fumes
  - Dust
  - Noise
  - Vibration
  - Waste/sewage
  - Radiation
  - Asbestos
  - Animals
- Consider duration and 'dose' of exposure – are symptoms worse towards the end of the day or when experiencing a higher exposure?
- Ask about exposure control, e.g. ventilation and personal protective clothing
- Consider whether the patient's symptoms improve over the weekend or when they go on holiday
- Consider asking if any of their colleagues have had similar symptoms/issues

Asbestos-related disease

- Wide spectrum of disease presentations, including
  - Pleural plaques
  - Pleural thickening
  - Asbestosis
  - Asbestos-related benign pleural effusion
  - Lung cancer
  - Malignant mesothelioma
- Patients may be eligible for compensation if they can demonstrate that their disease is likely due to an occupational exposure for which they did not receive adequate protection

Mrs North says that she used to work as a decorator for a large company who renovated old buildings to repurpose them as office space. She knows that she was exposed to asbestos and dust at this time, around 30 years ago. She doesn't recall using any protective equipment or taking any particular precautions at the time because 'it wasn't the done thing in those days'.

Mrs North goes for her CT after lunch. See Figures 17.3 and 17.4.

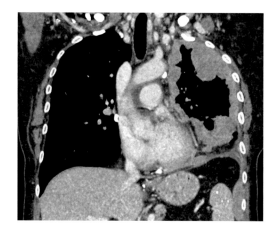

Figure 17.3 Coronal post-contrast CT image of the chest.

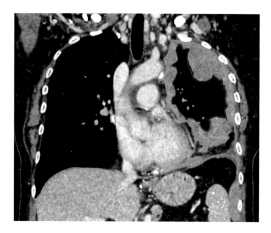

Figure 17.4 The same coronal CT image (Figure 17.3) with key features highlighted. The blue outline indicates the volume loss of the left hemithorax, compared to the right. The red outline delineates the abnormal pleural soft tissue. The green outline highlights the presence of calcified pleural plaques. Overall, appearances are in keeping with mesothelioma, likely due to previous asbestos exposure.

The junior doctor checks the report in the middle of the afternoon.

Volume loss seen in the left hemithorax compared to the right. Abnormal pleural soft tissue noted with the presence of calcified pleural plaques. Likely consistent with mesothelioma. There is a 9 mm hypodense lesion in segment VI of the liver suspicious for metastatic deposit. Multiple small bilateral pulmonary nodules (2 mm to 5.5 mm) which are suspicious in appearance. There is a mixed sclerotic and lytic lesion in the inferior pubic ramus and several sclerotic foci in the right ilium.

Conclusion: Probable mesothelioma with lesions suspicious for metastasis in the lungs and bones.

The junior doctor shows the report to the respiratory consultant, who goes to explain the results to Mrs North.

What should be considered when breaking the news to the patient?

There are many techniques and frameworks for this.

Key points

- Preparation
  - Find a quiet and private location
  - Avoid giving bad news over the phone if possible
  - Consider whether the patient may want a friend or family member present
  - Turn off bleeps and mobile phones
  - Consider booking a double appointment if in a clinic setting
  - Ensure that you have read through the notes and are familiar with all of the facts
- Communication
  - Establish what patient already knows
  - Avoid jargon and abbreviations
  - Pause to check understanding
  - Give a warning shot before breaking the news
  - Consider how much detail the patient may or may not wish to know – follow patient cues
  - Reassure without providing false hope
- Closing
  - Explain next steps
  - Arrange appropriate follow-up, e.g. with specialist nurses
  - Give written material if possible

Given the presence of bone metastases, the consultant asks the junior doctor to add on a calcium level to the morning bloods.

TIMEPOINT ⏱ 3

Later that day, the junior doctor on the ward is chasing up Mrs North's blood test results. Her calcium comes back as 3.4 mmol/L.

What are the causes of hypercalcaemia?

- Primary hyperparathyroidism

- Malignancy
  - Related to malignancy directly
    - Ectopic PTH, calcitriol or parathyroid hormone-related peptide production
  - Related to bone metastasis
    - Uncommon but can occur with mesothelioma
    - More common tumours to metastasise to bone include lung, breast, renal and myeloma
- Medication-induced, e.g. thiazide diuretics, lithium
- Rhabdomyolysis
- Thyrotoxicosis
- Phaeochromocytoma
- Primary adrenal insufficiency
- Sarcoidosis
- Tuberculosis
- Tertiary hyperparathyroidism

Approximately 90% of cases of hypercalcaemia are due to either primary hyperparathyroidism or malignancy.

What are the symptoms of hypercalcaemia?

- Nausea and vomiting
- Polyuria
- Low mood and confusion
- Weakness
- Abdominal pain
- Arrhythmias (shortened QTc)
- Drowsiness
- Constipation

How should hypercalcaemia be managed?

- Check renal function, liver function, thyroid function, myeloma screen, phosphate levels and parathyroid hormone levels to look for an underlying cause. Assess fluid balance and perform an ECG
- Rehydration with 0.9% sodium chloride
  - Give 4–6 litres over 24 hours
  - Consider giving loop diuretics if fluid overload (monitor elderly patients or

Table 17.1 Examples of anticipatory medications and sample doses

Symptom	Medication	Sample subcutaneous PRN dose	Sample syringe driver dose (continuous subcutaneous infusion/CSCI)
Pain (opioid-naïve)	Morphine sulphate	2.5–5 mg 2–4 hourly	10–20 mg/24 hours
Pain (already using morphine)	Morphine sulphate	Divide total daily oral morphine dose by **12** e.g. current dose 30 mg MST BD = 60 mg per day 60 ÷ 12 = 5 mg 2–4 hourly	Divide total daily oral morphine dose by **2** e.g. current dose 30 mg MST BD = 60 mg per day 60 ÷ 2 = 30 mg over 24 hours
Breathlessness	Midazolam	2.5 mg 2–4 hourly	10–20 mg/24 hours
Nausea	Cyclizine	50 mg 8 hourly	100–150 mg/24 hours
Secretions	Glycopyrronium bromide	0.2 mg 6 hourly	0.6–1.2 mg/24 hours
Anxiety and agitation	Midazolam	2.5–5 mg 2 hourly	10–20 mg/24 hours
Delirium and agitation	Haloperidol	1.5–3 mg 2 hourly	1.5–10 mg/24 hours

those with renal impairment carefully). Consider need for dialysis if severe renal impairment

- Intravenous bisphosphonates
  - Give *after* rehydration
  - Take 2–4 days to reach full effect
  - Options
    - Zoledronic acid 4 mg over 15 minutes
    - Pamidronate 30–90 mg at 20 mg/hour
    - Ibandronic acid 2–4 mg
- Second-line treatments include prednisolone, calcitonin and cinacalcet. Parathyroidectomy may be required in severe acute primary hyperparathyroidism

TIMEPOINT 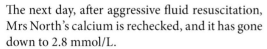 4

The next day, after aggressive fluid resuscitation, Mrs North's calcium is rechecked, and it has gone down to 2.8 mmol/L.

Mrs North is reviewed by the oncology consultant and palliative care specialist nurse on the ward in the afternoon. The consultant explains that due to her extensive disease, unfortunately active management would not be appropriate. After a long and difficult discussion, Mrs North agrees not to undergo any further active treatment. The palliative nurse suggests that she consider going to a hospice for symptom control as she is still requiring significant input to manage her breathlessness. Mrs North agrees to this.

What medications should be prescribed for a palliative discharge?

'Just in case' or 'anticipatory' medications may be given in hospital to patients nearing the end of life to help with symptom management. Patients may also be given the medications to go home with (to be administered by a district nurse) or if they are going to a hospice as a palliative discharge. These medications can be given subcutaneously when needed or through a syringe driver. Most trusts will have a guideline regarding their preferred choices for anticipatory prescribing, but Table 17.1 summarises some of the common medications used and their doses. Remember that elderly or frail patients, or patients with renal or liver impairment, may require reduced doses.

Mrs North is discharged to the local hospice. She passes away 2 weeks later. The hospice doctor is called to confirm her death.

What is the process for confirming the death of a patient?

- Confirm the identity of the patient by checking their wristband
- Observe for signs of life throughout
- Check for a response to verbal and painful stimulus
- Check the appearance of the pupils (dilated and fixed with no response to light)
- Assess for 3 minutes in total for the presence of
  - Respiratory sounds on auscultation
  - Heart sounds on auscultation
  - Carotid or other central pulse
- It is good practice to palpate for a pacemaker as these need to be removed if the patient has requested to be cremated
- Document the time and date of death
- If possible, document who was present at time of death
- Include your name, designation and GMC number

Case 18

TIMEPOINT 🕐 1

Mrs Moloney is a 64-year-old cleaner who presents to the emergency department as she has been feeling unwell all week, and when she checked her temperature at home had a fever of 38.7°C. She has had a cough and shortness of breath for 6 days and was started on antibiotics for a presumed chest infection by her GP 4 days ago. However, she feels that her condition has been deteriorating despite the antibiotics, and she has now started coughing up thick green sputum. She denies chest pain, weight loss and haemoptysis.

Her only past medical history is type 2 diabetes, for which she takes metformin 1 g BD. She has never smoked and drinks only 1 or 2 small glasses of wine a night. She spent a week in Spain around 8 months ago, but has not travelled since then.

Mrs Moloney has already been put on 24% oxygen by the triage nurse.

Her observations show:

Respiratory rate: 24/min
Oxygen saturations: 97% on 24% oxygen
Temperature: 38.4°C
Blood pressure: 132/59 mmHg
Heart rate: 88 bpm

Her heart sounds are normal, but she has decreased expansion over the right hemithorax, with a stony dull percussion note, reduced breath sounds and reduced vocal resonance at the right base. Abdominal and neurological examination are unremarkable.

The emergency doctor is concerned that Mrs Moloney may have developed a pleural effusion as a result of a chest infection.

What investigations should be arranged at this stage?

- Bloods
  - FBC – infection, anaemia
  - U&Es – baseline cause of effusion
  - CRP – infection
  - LFTs – atypical pneumonia, liver failure as cause of effusion
  - BNP – heart failure
- Chest X-ray

Initial blood test results are given in Table 18.1.

The chest radiograph shows a moderate-sized, right-sided pleural effusion.

Table 18.1 Venous blood tests

Haemoglobin	126 g/L
White cell count	14.3×10^9/L
Neutrophils	11.2×10^9/L
Lymphocytes	1.4×10^9/L
Platelets	464×10^9/L
Sodium	136 mmol/L
Potassium	3.9 mmol/L
Urea	7.4 mmol/L
Creatinine	87 µmol/L
Bilirubin	13 µmol/L
ALT	29 U/L
AST	26 U/L
Albumin	37 g/L
Protein	72 g/L
Glucose	5.9 mmol/L
CRP	112 mg/L
LDH	210 U/L

DOI: 10.1201/9781351257725-18

In light of the initial investigation findings, what further investigations should be arranged?

An ultrasound-guided pleural aspiration should be arranged. It is important to check that the patient has a normal clotting profile first.

When sending a pleural aspiration, what tests should be requested?

Samples should be sent for the following:

- Biochemistry: protein, LDH, glucose, lactate
- Microbiology: MC&S, acid fast bacilli staining and culture
- pH
- Cytology

In some hospitals, it is possible to check glucose, lactate and pH on a blood gas analyser to get instant point of care results.

TIMEPOINT ⏱ 2

Two hours later, Mrs Moloney has been admitted to the ward. The ward doctor is able to see some of the preliminary results which are available from the pleural aspiration.

Results of pleural aspiration

Protein	44 g/L
LDH	315 U/L
Glucose	3.1 mmol/L
pH	7.42

Into which two categories can pleural effusions be divided? Discuss the criteria used to distinguish between the categories.

Pleural effusions can be divided into transudates and exudates using Light's criteria.

Pleural fluid is considered to be exudative if it meets any of the following criteria:

- Pleural fluid protein/serum protein ratio >0.5
- Pleural fluid LDH/serum LDH ratio >0.6
- Pleural fluid LDH >2/3 of the upper limit of normal for serum LDH

Transudates are caused by decreased oncotic pressure or increased hydrostatic pressure. Common causes of transudates are left ventricular failure, nephrotic syndrome and liver cirrhosis. Exudates are caused by increased capillary permeability. Common causes of exudates are infections, malignancy and connective tissue disease.

How should Mrs Moloney be managed?

Mrs Moloney's pleural effusion is an exudate, with a history and test results suggestive of a parapneumonic effusion. She therefore requires appropriate antibiotic treatment.

The ward doctor starts Mrs Moloney on IV co-amoxiclav 1.2 g TDS and oral clarithromycin 500 mg BD, in accordance with local microbiology guidelines.

TIMEPOINT ⏱ 3

Five days after admission, the ward doctor is called to see Mrs Moloney as she is spiking a temperature of 39.2°C, despite having taken 4 days of intravenous antibiotics. She asks the nurse to repeat her observations.

Her observations show:

Respiratory rate: 28/min
Oxygen saturations: 94% on 2 L oxygen via nasal cannulae
Temperature: 39.2°C
Blood pressure: 104/75 mmHg
Heart rate: 124 bpm

On examination, she still has a dull-sounding right base with coarse crackles in the midzone.

The doctor requests a repeat chest X-ray. See Figures 18.1 and 18.2.

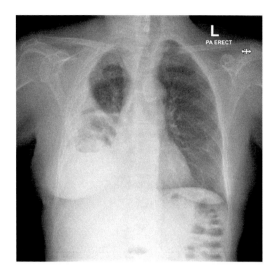

Figure 18.1 The chest X-ray shows a right sided pleural effusion, which appears more complex; suggestive of an empyema.

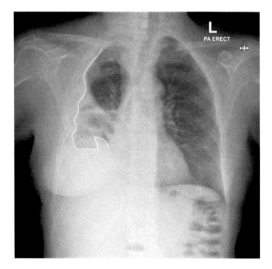

Figure 18.2 The white outline on the same image (Figure 18.1) demarcates the loculated nature of the effusion. Generally, empyemas tend to form a lenticular shape (biconvex) against the chest wall.

After viewing the results, the ward doctor calls the on-call respiratory registrar who agrees to help with a pleural aspiration. Thick, cloudy fluid is aspirated from the pleural space under ultrasound guidance.

Later that evening, the microbiology lab phones through to the ward to inform them that pus cells have been seen in Mrs Moloney's pleural fluid.

What is the diagnosis, and how should Mrs Moloney be managed?

Pus cells in the pleural fluid are indicative of an empyema. Empyema has a 15% mortality rate, so senior-led management is important. The pus needs to be drained from the pleural space. This can often be done with a chest drain, but up to 30% require surgical drainage via thoracoscopy (VATS). The case should be discussed with a thoracic surgeon. VATS has no mortality benefit over simple chest drain insertion, but does reduce length of admission. CT imaging will allow a better assessment of the degree of loculation, and will inform the decision as to whether to manage with VATS. The evidence suggests that flushing the chest drain with fibrinolytics does not improve the outcome.

Appropriate antibiotic therapy should be discussed with a microbiologist and should be guided by microscopy, culture and sensitivity of the pleural fluid. The organism responsible for the empyema is usually the same organism responsible for the pneumonia, and knowledge of local conditions should guide empiric treatment. Aminoglycosides (e.g. gentamicin, streptomycin) are not effective at low pH and should not be used. Duration of antibiotic therapy should be guided by the identity of the organism and its sensitivities, and by clinical response. Often 4–6 weeks is recommended.

TIMEPOINT ⏱ 4

Two hours later, the night-shift medical registrar receives a handover from the day team that an urgent chest drain is required for an empyema. Unfortunately, it was not done during the evening shift as the team was busy attending to a peri-arrest patient.

The medical registrar prepares their equipment for the chest drain and consents Mrs Moloney.

What are the complications of chest drain insertion?

- Pain
- Failed procedure (incorrectly sited)
- Bleeding
- Infection
- Pneumothorax
- Haemothorax
- Damage to intercostal nerve
- Pulmonary oedema
- Organ damage

The registrar explains the procedure, including the risks and benefits, and answers all of Mrs Moloney's questions. She agrees to go ahead with the procedure.

The registrar sets up his sterile field, cleans the area for insertion and gives local anaesthetic. He then inserts the needle into the pleural space and advances the guidewire. He makes a small incision and then passes the dilator over the guidewire, and then finally passes the chest drain over the guidewire. As soon as the tubing is connected, frank blood is seen in the tubing. The blood pressure machine shows 78/43 mmHg. The tube continues to drain blood and Mrs Moloney stops responding. The doctor pulls the emergency buzzer and a nurse quickly runs in with a crash trolley. The healthcare assistant puts out a crash call whilst the registrar and the nurse commence advanced life support.

What reversible causes should be considered during advanced life support? What are the likely causes in this case?

The causes can be summarised as the 4 Hs and the 4 Ts.

- Hypoxia
- Hypovolaemia
- Hypokalaemia/hyperkalaemia/other metabolic derangement
- Hypothermia
- Toxins
- Tension pneumothorax
- Tamponade (cardiac)
- Thrombosis (coronary or pulmonary)

The likely causes in this scenario are either a cardiac tamponade or a hypovolaemic arrest.

The rest of the crash team arrive and continue advanced life support. A bedside ultrasound scan shows no evidence of tamponade, so Mrs Moloney is treated as a hypovolaemic arrest secondary to iatrogenic large vessel trauma from the chest drain insertion. Unfortunately, despite the best efforts of the team, they are unable to resuscitate Mrs Moloney, and after six cycles the decision is made to stop.

FURTHER READING

1. Case study with parallels to Timepoint 4: Vignau Cano J.M., Bermúdez García A., Macías Rubio D. Lesión de aorta torácica por tubo pleural. *Med Intensiva.* 2019;43:192. DOI: 10.1016/j.medine.2019.01.005

Case 19

TIMEPOINT ⏱ 1

Mr Williams is a 58-year-old plumber who attends his GP complaining of a cough. He is starting to worry that the cough has been going on for too long which is why he has presented today. He guesses that it has been going on for at least 6 months now, but probably less than a year. The cough is sometimes productive, but the sputum is always clear. He denies being breathless at rest, although he admits that he is increasingly breathless on exertion which is starting to interfere with his work. He also struggles to keep up with his wife when they are out walking. He denies having any chest pain, any difficulty sleeping due to breathlessness or any weight loss. He has never coughed up any blood.

In terms of past medical history, Mr Williams has well-controlled hypertension. He has also had adhesive capsulitis of the left shoulder in the past, and a right-sided Colles' fracture many years ago. The GP notes that over the last few years Mr Williams has seemed to present recurrently in the winter months with respiratory tract infections and has received numerous courses of antibiotics for these. He takes ramipril 5 mg daily, and has no allergies that he is aware of. He drinks a couple of pints of lager each evening at the pub, and smokes around 30–40 cigarettes a day. He says that he has been smoking for 40 odd years now so is really struggling to cut down, although he knows that he should.

On examination he appears well, with no obvious signs of respiratory distress.

His observations are:

Respiratory rate: 22/min
Oxygen saturations: 94% on room air

Temperature: 36.6°C
Blood pressure: 129/85 mmHg
Heart rate: 84 bpm

On examination, he is warm and well perfused peripherally with a capillary refill time of less than 2 seconds and no evidence of cyanosis. His pulse is approximately 80 beats per minute and regular. His JVP is not raised. His trachea is central with a reduced cricosternal distance. On auscultation, wheezing can be heard throughout the lung fields, but no crepitations. There is no evidence of sacral or pedal oedema.

The GP wonders if COPD might be a good explanation for Mr Williams' symptoms, given his extensive smoking history.

What initial investigations should be carried out if COPD is suspected?

- Calculation of BMI
- Full blood count to assess for anaemia or polycythaemia
- Chest X-ray to exclude other lung pathologies
- Spirometry, including post-bronchodilator testing, should be performed at diagnosis
- Sputum culture should be considered in order to identify organisms if sputum is purulent
- Serial peak flow measurements should be considered in order to exclude asthma if there is still uncertainty regarding the diagnosis
- ECG, BNP and echo should be considered if there is a history of cardiovascular disease or features of pulmonary hypertension
- Serum alpha-1 antitrypsin should be considered if the patient is younger than 35 years, or has a minimal smoking history, or has a family history of lung disease

What advice could Mr Williams be given regarding smoking cessation, irrespective of his spirometry results?

- Smoking cessation is a key element of lifestyle management of COPD
- Patients with COPD should be offered smoking cessation advice at every healthcare contact
- This may include brief advice, behavioural support, nicotine replacement therapy, varenicline or bupropion if needed
- Current evidence suggests that e-cigarettes are significantly less dangerous than smoking but are not completely risk-free, and the long-term impact of their use is still unknown
- If a patient is not yet ready to stop smoking, remind them again of the benefits of stopping and encourage them to seek help in the future when they feel more ready

The GP discusses smoking cessation with Mr Williams, and he agrees to try a course of varenicline and referral to a behavioural support programme. She prescribes him a salbutamol inhaler to use as required, and refers him for spirometry at the local hospital. She also requests that he be assessed for pulmonary rehabilitation.

TIMEPOINT ⏱ 2

One week later, the GP reviews Mr Williams' spirometry results.

What would you expect to see on spirometry?

You would expect to see evidence of obstructive airway disease, defined as a post-bronchodilator FEV1/FVC <0.7. Severity can then be stratified using the FEV1 as a percentage of the predicted value.

Spirometry is an important tool both for diagnosis but also for the monitoring of disease progression. Although the level of airway obstruction does not correlate well with the extent of the patient's disability, it helps to guide treatment and estimate prognosis.

Spirometry demonstrates an FEV1/FVC of 0.63 and FEV1 58% of predicted.

The GP phones Mr Williams to ask him how he is getting on. He reports that he does not think the blue inhaler has helped him very much. He has been using it 6–7 times a day when he feels breathless on exertion, but it doesn't seem to make much difference. The GP explains that the spirometry confirms a diagnosis of COPD, and suggests starting a LAMA-LABA inhaler. She also asks him to book an appointment for influenza and pneumococcal vaccinations. Mr Williams is happy with this plan.

How should inhalers be escalated (Figure 19.1)?

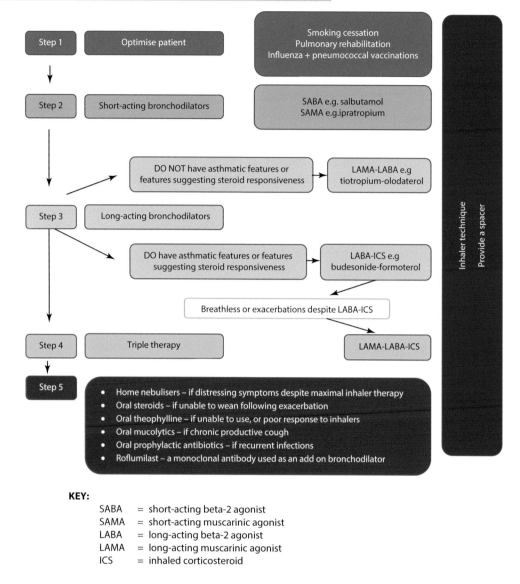

Figure 19.1 Escalation of treatment in COPD.

KEY:

SABA = short-acting beta-2 agonist
SAMA = short-acting muscarinic agonist
LABA = long-acting beta-2 agonist
LAMA = long-acting muscarinic agonist
ICS = inhaled corticosteroid

Surgical options for severe COPD

- Lung volume reduction
- Bullectomy
- Lung transplant

How can COPD be staged?

Either using post-bronchodilatory FEV1 (GOLD scale) (Table 19.1) or using the MRC dyspnoea scale (Table 19.2).

Table 19.1 GOLD scale for COPD staging

Stage	Description	FEV1
1	Mild	≥80% predicted
2	Moderate	50–79% predicted
3	Severe	30–49% predicted
4	Very severe	<30% predicted

Table 19.2 MRC dyspnoea scale

Grade	Degree of breathlessness
1	Only breathless with strenuous exercise
2	Breathless when hurrying or walking up a slight hill
3	Walks slower than peers on flat ground due to breathlessness Has to stop for breath when walking at own pace
4	Stops for breath after walking for a few minutes on flat ground Stops for breath after walking approximately 100 metres
5	Housebound due to breathlessness Breathless when dressing or undressing

TIMEPOINT ⏲ 3

Three months later, Mr Williams presents to the emergency department as he is feeling unwell. Over the last 3 days he has been feeling increasingly short of breath, to the point that he is now quite significantly short of breath at rest. He has also been coughing much more than usual and has noticed that his sputum has turned yellow-green in colour. He generally feels run down and exhausted and has not been to work the last couple of days.

His observations are:

Respiratory rate: 26/min
Oxygen saturations: 95% on room air
Temperature: 38.4°C
Blood pressure: 134/91 mmHg
Heart rate: 99 bpm

On examination he appears to be moderately breathless at rest and is using his accessory muscles to breathe. He is not obviously cyanosed. He continues to cough throughout the examination and has an expiratory wheeze that is audible from the end of the bed. He appears to have a fine tremor. The trachea is central. Percussion of the lung fields is normal.

On auscultation, there are coarse crepitations in the right midzone with loud wheeze throughout the lung fields. There is no peripheral oedema.

The emergency department doctor is concerned that this deterioration may represent an infective exacerbation of his COPD.

What are the common causes of infective exacerbations of COPD?

- Bacterial, e.g. *Streptococcus pneumoniae, Haemophilus influenzae, Moraxella catarrhalis, Staphylococcus aureus, Pseudomonas aeruginosa*
- Viral, e.g. rhinovirus, influenza, parainfluenza, respiratory syncytial virus, adenovirus, coronavirus

How should an infective exacerbation of COPD be investigated and managed?

- Investigations
  - Bedside
    - Sputum culture – to guide antibiotic choices if sensitivities are available
    - ECG – evidence of right heart strain
  - Blood tests
    - Full blood count and CRP – markers of infection may be raised
    - U&E and LFT – may affect medications prescribed
    - Theophylline levels – important if patient is on theophylline as a narrow therapeutic window
    - Blood cultures – evidence of bacteraemia
    - ABG – evidence of carbon dioxide retention or respiratory failure, to help guide oxygen prescription
  - Imaging
    - Chest X-ray – evidence of consolidation or another pathology

- Management
  - Regular salbutamol and/or ipratropium inhalers or nebulisers. **Nebulisers may need to be driven by air rather than oxygen if evidence of hypercapnia**
  - Oral prednisolone 30 mg for 7–14 days
  - Antibiotics as per local guidelines/available sensitivities if purulent sputum or consolidation on chest X-ray

Mr Williams provides blood and sputum samples which are sent to the lab. His ECG is unremarkable, and his initial ABG is within normal parameters except for a mildly raised bicarbonate. The doctor does not start oxygen as his saturations seem to be reasonable. Mr Williams is started on regular nebulisers to manage his symptoms and goes for a chest X-ray when the porter is available. The emergency department doctor reviews the X-ray and sees evidence of consolidation, so starts him on the treatment for an infective exacerbation of COPD, including prednisolone, co-amoxiclav and doxycycline.

Shortly after this he is moved to the acute medical unit. Later in the evening, the nurse repeats Mr Williams' observations.

His observations are:

Respiratory rate: 32/min
Saturations: 86% on room air
Temperature: 38.2°C
Blood pressure: 142/95 mmHg
Heart rate: 113 bpm

She is concerned about his NEWS score of 9 and calls the on-call doctor, who attends and repeats Mr Williams' ABG (Table 19.3).

Table 19.3 Arterial blood gas results

	Previous ABG	Current ABG
pH	7.41	7.29
PCO_2	5.8 kPa	7.7 kPa
PO_2	8.9 kPa	7.1 kPa
HCO_3	26.2 mmol/L	27.6 mmol/L
Base excess	1.4 mmol/L	0.7 mmol/L
Lactate	1.6 mmol/L	1.5 mmol/L

When should non-invasive ventilation (NIV) be started, and what should be done prior to starting?

- If the following are still present after 60 minutes, despite optimising medical therapy (including target oxygen saturations of 88–92%)
  - pH <7.35
  - PCO_2 >6.5 kPa
  - Respiratory rate >23 breaths/minute
- An ABG should always be performed prior to starting NIV to confirm the above parameters
- It is recommended to perform a chest X-ray but this should not delay starting NIV if the patient is deteriorating
- The patient should be investigated for reversible causes of respiratory failure, and these should be treated
- A treatment escalation plan should be in place before NIV is started so that there is a plan in the event of NIV failing
- Consideration should be given to whether invasive ventilation might be more appropriate – if this is the case, it is not essential to trial NIV first
- Consider stopping or weaning NIV when pH and PCO_2 have normalised

The on-call doctor discusses the situation with the medical registrar, who agrees that it would be appropriate to trial NIV for Mr Williams. Mr Williams is moved to the respiratory support unit where he is started on NIV. He responds well to this, and so it is continued for 72 hours before being weaned off. He also continues to receive the rest of the treatment that he was started on. Once the NIV is stopped, he remains under the respiratory team for another 2 days before being discharged home.

TIMEPOINT 🕐 4

Nine months later, Mr Williams attends his GP for his first annual COPD review. He has been stable since his infective exacerbation 9 months back and has not needed to be admitted to hospital again. Overall his exercise tolerance has improved compared to before he started any treatment, and he is managing well at work. He is not breathless at rest. He still coughs sometimes but not as much as previously. He is still smoking, but has managed to cut down to around 15 cigarettes a day, and is aiming to cut down further still. His inhaler technique is good and he is compliant with his current inhalers. The GP checks his oxygen saturations, which are 94%, and the rest of his cardiovascular and respiratory examination is unremarkable. The GP also notes a recent full blood count which was normal.

He has recently had his spirometry re-tested which demonstrates an FEV1/FVC of 0.61 and FEV1 53% of predicted. The GP asks about how breathless Mr Williams is day-to-day. Mr Williams reports that he now only becomes breathless when he is rushing or walking up hills or stairs. The GP is pleased that his disease seems to be stable and that symptomatically he has improved since his diagnosis.

Mr Williams has recently joined a local COPD support group. The friends he has made there have encouraged him to research more about his COPD, to allow him to make informed decisions about his treatment. He has been doing some research on the Internet and wants to know if he would benefit from long-term oxygen therapy (LTOT), as he has friends who say that it has made a huge difference to them.

The GP says that he does not think his COPD is severe enough for him to qualify.

Who should be assessed, and what are the criteria for starting long-term oxygen therapy (LTOT)?

Patients with stable COPD who are receiving optimum medical management may benefit from LTOT. They should be non-smokers due to the risk of explosion if they smoke near the oxygen concentrators.

COPD patients with the following should be assessed for starting LTOT:

- Very severe or severe airflow obstruction (FEV1 ≤49% of predicted)
- Cyanosis, peripheral oedema or a raised JVP

- Oxygen saturations ≤92% on room air
- Polycythaemia

Patients who qualify for assessment should have two ABGs taken at least 3 weeks apart.

LTOT may be offered to patients with:

- PaO_2 <7.3 kPa
- PaO_2 between 7.3 kPa and 8.0 kPa with one or more of the following
  - Peripheral oedema
  - Pulmonary hypertension
  - Secondary polycythaemia

Patients need to use the oxygen for at least 15 hours a day to derive a survival benefit. They are likely to require the oxygen lifelong.

Ambulatory oxygen therapy may be considered for patients on LTOT who wish to use oxygen therapy outside the home, or patients not requiring LTOT but who have exercise desaturation.

Mr Williams thanks the GP for the explanation. He then asks about whether he should be started on long-term antibiotics, as he has met some friends who are on regular antibiotics to stop them from getting chest infections.

When should prophylactic antibiotics be started, and which drug is recommended?

Prophylactic antibiotics should be considered in patients who:

- Have frequent (≥4/year) exacerbations
- Have prolonged exacerbations
- Have exacerbations resulting in hospitalisation

Prior to starting antibiotics, patients should have stopped smoking, have completed pulmonary rehabilitation, have been vaccinated appropriately and have optimised inhaled management. They should also have sputum cultures sent and a CT thorax to rule out other lung pathologies. The patient should also be trained in airway clearance techniques.

The recommended antibiotic is azithromycin 250 mg, 3 times per week. Before starting this the patient should have an ECG to check for a long QT interval, and baseline LFTs.

Mr Williams feels that as he has only had one exacerbation of COPD this year, he would like to hold off starting antibiotics for now. The GP agrees with him, but warns him that there is a reasonable chance he may need to start antibiotics at some point in the future. Overall the GP is pleased that Mr Williams' COPD is reasonably stable. The GP encourages Mr Williams to continue to cut down on his smoking, and reminds him to come back sooner than the next annual review if there is any deterioration in his symptoms.

Case 20

Mr Shabbs is a 67-year-old retired metal work engineering executive. He likes hill walking and had experienced little difficulty doing so until 18 months ago when he became progressively breathless on what he regarded as less difficult slopes in Scotland. He presents to his GP as the reduced exercise tolerance has gradually progressed, and now he feels short of breath walking just 20 metres. He had been treated for depression on two different occasions in his 40s; otherwise he has no past medical history. He lives with his wife and has three adult sons. He is on no medication and has no allergies. He's never smoked and rarely drinks alcohol. His observations are:

Respiratory rate: 22/min
Oxygen saturations: 91% on room air
Temperature: 36.7°C
Blood pressure: 130/80 mmHg
Heart rate: 94 bpm

On examination, Mr Shabbs has finger clubbing and lower zone fine inspiratory crepitations.

The GP feels the clinical picture is suggestive of a fibrotic lung disease and makes an urgent respiratory referral incorporating a request for lung function testing.

What are the causes of clubbing?

See Table 20.1.

TIMEPOINT ⏲ 2

Three weeks later, Mr Shabbs is seen at a chest clinic. The clinic has a one-stop new diagnosis system whereby core investigations can be set up to take place prior to the afternoon clinic consultation. His observations are:

Respiratory rate: 20/min
Oxygen saturations: 92% on room air
Temperature: 36.5°C
Blood pressure: 132/70 mmHg
Heart rate: 92 bpm

What investigations should be done next?

1. Antibodies; ANA/ANCA/Anti GBM/ AntiScl-70/ ENA
2. High-resolution CT chest

These results show:

1. Antibodies are all normal/negative
2. High-resolution CT chest (Figure 20.1) – this is abnormal and entirely consistent with an idiopathic pulmonary fibrosis picture incorporating honeycombing >25%, fibrosis score >30% and traction bronchiectasis

The clinic concludes with a plan to have a multidisciplinary meeting in the very near future to discuss the treatment options for Mr Shabbs, based on a working diagnosis of interstitial lung disease (ILD); likely idiopathic pulmonary fibrosis (IPF).

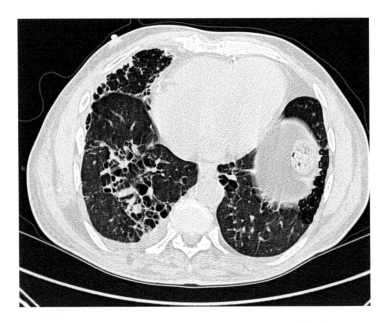

Figure 20.1 High resolution computed tomography (HRCT) axial image demonstrating subpleural 'honeycomb' change, which is characteristic of usual interstitial pneumonitis (UIP). UIP is the hallmark of idiopathic pulmonary fibrosis. There are layers of thick-walled, irregular cysts replacing normal lung parenchyma (red outline).

What are the more recent treatment options in ILD/IPF?

There are two new agents whose mechanism of action suggests promising potential for efficacy to treat these conditions; nintedanib and pirfenidone. Nintedanib inhibits tyrosine kinase receptors and thus seems to interfere with vascular endothelial growth factor (VEGF) and fibroblast growth factor action thus reducing fibrosis. Pirfenidone appears to have anti-inflammatory and fibrotic-reducing activity.

TIMEPOINT ⏲ 3

Two months later, Mr Shabbs was seen for a further chest clinic review after he had been trialled on both of the above medications (each for around a month). Unfortunately he feels that neither of them made a huge difference. He had simply tried to gently enjoy the fresh air and take slow gentle strolls in the local park, but was very breathless even after those.

On clinical review, observations are as follows:

Respiratory rate: 20/min
Oxygen saturations: 87% on room air
Temperature: 36.7°C
Blood pressure: 131/81 mmHg
Heart rate: 88 bpm

Over the following months, Mr Shabbs has found it increasingly difficult to walk around the house and perform activities of daily living. Specialist physiotherapy and occupational therapy were involved. He was advised to join a support group.

What is the role of support groups in chronic disease?

There is an enormous array of international, national and local medical support groups that are crucial for campaigning and supporting the needs of certain medical conditions. In the fields

Table 20.1 Causes of clubbing

Primary	Primary hypertrophic osteoarthropathy
	Familial clubbing
Pulmonary disease	Lung cancer
	Tuberculosis
	Bronchiectasis
	Cystic fibrosis
	Interstitial lung disease
	Idiopathic pulmonary fibrosis
	Sarcoidosis
	Lipoid pneumonia
	Empyema
	Pleural mesothelioma
	Pulmonary artery sarcoma
	Cryptogenic fibrosing alveolitis
	Pulmonary metastases
Cardiac disease	Cyanotic congenital heart disease
	Other causes of right-to-left shunting
	Bacterial endocarditis
Gastrointestinal disease	Ulcerative colitis
	Crohn's disease
	Primary biliary cirrhosis
	Cirrhosis of the liver
	Leiomyoma of the oesophagus
	Achalasia
	Peptic ulceration of the oesophagus
Skin disease	Bureau–Barrière–Thomas syndrome (digital clubbing associated with palmoplantar keratoderma)
	Fischer's syndrome (keratosis palmaris et plantaris, hair hypoplasia, onycholysis and onychogryphosis)
	Palmoplantar keratoderma (diffuse patches on the palms and soles)
Malignancies	Thyroid cancer
	Thymus cancer
	Hodgkin's disease
	Disseminated chronic myeloid leukaemia (POEMS syndrome – polyneuropathy, organomegaly, endocrinopathy, monoclonal gammopathy and skin changes)
Miscellaneous conditions	Acromegaly
	Thyroid acropachy (clubbing associated with Graves' disease and periosteal new bone formation)
	Pregnancy

of chronic diseases, the ability to communicate through social media, provide magazines, open helplines and give practical support and political influence have enabled these groups to flourish. Examples of such organisations in the United Kingdom include Diabetes UK, MS Society, Asthma UK, the British Lung Foundation and Action for Pulmonary Fibrosis.

TIMEPOINT ⏱ 4

Around 3 months later, Mr Shabbs had used all the available support, multidisciplinary input, Web-based patient groups and medical treatment options available, but despite intense adherence to all recommended interventions, his condition inexorably progressed. The severity of the burden upon his life and his loved ones, plus the almost exhaustive use of active treatment options, meant that he and his specialist nurse started to discuss whether it might be worth considering a palliative care perspective.

Arrangements were made, and it was broadly agreed amongst all the relevant professionals that at this stage the prognosis was of relatively short duration; thus Mr Shabbs became increasingly familiar with the palliative care team, who he found were caring, sensitive and supportive.

What is known about the potential for palliative care in non-malignant disease?

In this case, and many other progressive or incurable conditions, there is international consensus that a palliative, kind, patient-centred approach to progressive non-malignant conditions can sometimes be considered. It all depends on the shared decision-making as to the prognosis and/or burden of the disease. Expertise has been developed in such scenarios, especially once life-sustaining treatment is either discontinued or not deemed to be appropriate. In particular, there is a wide recognition that this approach is increasingly needed for non-malignant diseases affecting the heart, lungs, kidneys and brain.

Particular examples include chronic respiratory disease, chronic kidney disease (when decisions are taken not to commence dialysis or to discontinue such treatment), chronic heart failure and progressive neurological conditions – such as rapidly advancing dementia and motor neuron disease. Commencement of palliative care can only start if everyone involved broadly agrees that Mr Shabbs might have entered into the last months/year of life. There is also a need for integrated care in terms of communication and liaison between primary- and secondary-care professionals. The revelation that the prognosis in some of such patients is worse than cancer and the progression of the disease is not always well-recognised. A relevant website is www.spict.org.uk.

FURTHER READING

1. Sgalla G, Iovene B, Calvello M, Ori M, Varone F, Richeldi L. Idiopathic pulmonary fibrosis: pathogenesis and management. *Respir Res.* 2018 Feb 22;19(1):32. doi: 10.1186/s12931-018-0730-2. Review.
2. Spicknall KE, Zirwas MJ, English JC 3rd Clubbing: an update on diagnosis, differential diagnosis, pathophysiology, and clinical relevance. *J Am Acad Dermatol.* 2005 Jun 52(6):1020–8.

Case 21

TIMEPOINT 1

Mrs Deane is a 76-year-old retired primary school teacher who has developed odd painful twinges in her right hip and groin over the last 4 months. She has a past history of acid reflux for which she uses omeprazole 20 mg daily, but is otherwise usually fit and well. She does not use any other medications and has no allergies.

Mrs Deane is usually able to walk comfortably 20 minutes to and from the supermarket, and do all of her other activities of daily living independently. She also attends Pilates and swimming classes weekly. However, her hip pain is now affecting her usual activities and in the last couple of weeks has started to disturb her sleep.

She attends her GP as she is still waking up with pain despite using paracetamol regularly, and occasionally ibuprofen when she is really struggling. She denies having had back pain, or pain in any of her other joints, and there is no history of trauma.

On examination, her basic observations are normal. The legs are of equal length. There is no obvious redness or swelling of the hip or knee, and there is no tenderness to palpation, including over the greater trochanter. She has a reasonable range of movement in the right hip, although this is less than her left hip. She has some discomfort on rotational movement.

Mrs Deane has never smoked and only drinks alcohol on Christmas Day. She was widowed when her husband passed away last year, after 53 years of marriage.

What is the most likely diagnosis?

In a 76-year-old woman with no trauma, the most likely diagnosis is osteoarthritis.

> The Oxford Hip Score may be used to assess patients with hip pain when osteoarthritis is suspected. It indicates whether conservative or surgical management is more likely to be appropriate.

The GP thinks that this may be osteoarthritis but is concerned that Mrs Deane is having pain at night, so arranges an X-ray of the pelvis. The GP suggests that Mrs Deane use the ibuprofen regularly (400 mg three times a day) and also prescribes codeine 30 mg for her to use if she has breakthrough pain.

Why might suggesting the use of regular ibuprofen be inappropriate for Mrs Deane?

NSAIDs have an increased risk of toxicity in the elderly. Common NSAID-related risks, including renal impairment, heart failure and gastrointestinal bleeding, are all more common in older adults. The BNF suggests that NSAIDs should be used cautiously in the elderly; for example, for ibuprofen, it states that there is a 'risk of serious side effects and fatalities' with systemic use. If it is necessary to give them, NSAIDs should ideally be given for the shortest possible length of time at the lowest possible dose.

TIMEPOINT 2

Two weeks later, Mrs Deane has her X-ray after returning from a beach holiday in Spain. The report is emailed urgently to her GP later that afternoon:

SIGNIFICANT ABNORMALITY ALERT: There is loss of the normal bony lines of the right acetabulum with a soap bubble appearance. The differentials include solitary bone lesions, both benign and malignant, and bony lesions from distant primary sites.

The GP telephones Mrs Deane and asks her to attend the surgery that evening to discuss the X-ray result. She explains that the X-ray report is very worrying, and that the worst-case scenario is that it could be cancer. On further questioning, the GP discovers that:

- Mrs Deane has lost about 6 kg in the last 6 months
- She does not have a cough and has never smoked
- Her bowel habit is normal
- She has no other systemic symptoms
- Mrs Deane's mother had breast cancer at the age of 60, as did two female cousins in their 60s
- Mrs Deane's sister had ovarian cancer diagnosed 2 years ago (at age 70)
- Mrs Deane attended breast screening at age 50 and 53 but found it very uncomfortable and did not attend after that

The GP gains consent to examine Mrs Deane's breasts.

Aside from a lump, what changes to the breast may be suggestive of breast cancer?

- A change in the size or shape of the breast
- A change to the nipple, e.g. rash, change in shape, inversion
- Nipple discharge
- Change in skin appearance, e.g. dimpling, puckering, rashes, peau d'orange
- Axillary lymphadenopathy
- Breast pain (uncommon)

On examination, the GP finds a hard, craggy, 4-cm lump in the right breast. There are also a couple of palpable right axillary nodes. The left breast and axilla are normal. The GP explains the findings to Mrs Deane and makes a 2-week wait referral to the breast clinic.

Other than a family history, what are the risk factors for breast cancer?

- Being female
- Increasing age
- Previous history of breast cancer
- Previous history of some other cancers including melanoma, lung cancer and endometrial cancer
- Nulliparity or first pregnancy after age 30
- Never breastfeeding
- Continuous combined HRT
- Dense breast tissue
- Early menarche
- Late menopause
- Being overweight after the age of menopause
- High alcohol intake
- Smoking
- Being inactive
- Diabetes mellitus
- Radiation to the chest area
- Combined oral contraceptive pill (however, the risk is no longer increased 10 years after stopping the pill)

The GP checks that Mrs Deane will have support at home on leaving the surgery with this bad news, and offers to book an appointment to see Mrs Deane with her daughter the following week.

TIMEPOINT ⏱ 3

Five days later, Mrs Deane is seen at the one-stop breast clinic. She is examined by the consultant, and then has a mammogram and a fine needle aspiration. The consultant explains that clinically, this is a very suspicious lump. He arranges for her to have an urgent CT chest, abdomen and pelvis and also requests a staging bone scan.

Mrs Deane asks the consultant if it was wrong that she was never put on a high-risk screening programme, given that her mother and two cousins had breast cancer. The consultant explains that only those who are known to have specific genetic mutations qualify for this. He goes on to explain that otherwise, only those with a very significant family history are seen by a specialist. Mrs Deane asks whether her 45-year-old daughter would be considered high risk.

According to the National Breast Cancer Screening Programme, which groups are considered high-risk and should be screened on the high-risk screening protocol?

The criteria for inclusion in the high-risk screening programme are limited, but include BRCA1 and BRCA2 carriers, patients with Li–Fraumeni syndrome and those who have had radiotherapy to the chest area below the age of 30.

However, NICE guidance suggests patients with any of the following should be referred to secondary care for further input:

- A first-degree female relative diagnosed with breast cancer aged under 40 years
- A first-degree male relative diagnosed with breast cancer at any age
- A first-degree relative with bilateral breast cancer under 50 years
- Two first-degree relatives, or one first- and one second-degree relatives with breast cancer at any age
- One first-degree or second-degree relative diagnosed with breast cancer at any age, and one first-degree or second-degree relative diagnosed with ovarian cancer at any age (one should be a first-degree relative)
- Three first-degree or second-degree relatives diagnosed with breast cancer at any age
- One first-degree or second-degree relative diagnosed over age 40, plus
  - Jewish ancestry
  - Sarcoma, glioma or other complicated patterns of multiple cancers
  - Two or more relatives with breast cancer on the father's side of the family

TIMEPOINT 🕐 4

One week later, the oncology consultant is reviewing all of Mrs Deane's results prior to her attending for another appointment. The CT scan shows metastatic deposits in the liver, and the bone scan shows lesions in the skull and ribs, as well as the right acetabulum, indicating a stage 4 cancer. The biopsy confirms a triple-negative histology. Mrs Deane is also found to be BRCA2 positive.

Mrs Deane also has a 39-year-old son. What would the potential risks be for him if he were BRCA2 positive as well?

- 5–10% lifetime breast cancer risk (0.1% in general population)
- 20–25% lifetime prostate cancer risk (11% in general population)
- 50% risk of passing gene on to children
- BRCA1 is much less significant in men

The consultant discusses the situation with Mrs Deane and her daughter, alongside the breast cancer specialist nurse. Mrs Deane feels strongly that she would not want any active treatment of her cancer if there is no cure, as she has seen friends suffer the side effects of treatment and 'wants to enjoy the time she has left'.

The consultant asks Mrs Deane what she is worried about. Mrs Deane says that she is most worried about her hip pain and how she will manage this. She asks what options there are available for treating her hip pain.

What are the options for the management of metastatic bone pain?

Bone is a common site for metastatic spread of cancers including prostate, lung, renal, breast and myeloma, and bone pain may cause significant morbidity; therefore knowledge of management options is important. The pain may be related to invasion of the bone itself, damage to the adjacent structures or pathological fractures.

Options include:

- Typical analgesics as per the WHO pain ladder
- External beam radiotherapy
  - Good response in around 50–80% of patients
  - Good option for single-site metastasis
  - May require multiple fractions
- Bisphosphonates or denosumab
  - Reduce incidence of fractures and hypercalcaemia and reduce the need for palliative radiotherapy or surgery
  - No reduction in the risk of spinal cord compression
- Stabilisation (e.g. bracing, collars) if complete or impending pathological fracture and not suitable for surgical intervention
- Local nerve blocks may be useful in some cases, e.g. rib metastases
- In some cancers, systemic anticancer treatments are important to help reduce metastatic pain

Mrs Deane's pain is well-controlled with external beam radiotherapy, and she has an excellent quality of life for the next few months. Sadly, her condition deteriorates, and she develops jaundice, more severe bone pain and loses more weight. She is prescribed oral nutritional supplements and morphine sulphate tablets. Her daughter moves in with her, and they have regular carers including Marie Curie nurses. As Mrs Deane finds swallowing more difficult and her pain is worsening, the GP visits and prescribes medications to be given via a syringe driver. The palliative care nurses administer this. Three months later, Mrs Deane passes away comfortably at home with her daughter present.

FURTHER READING

1. www.orthopaedicscore.com/scorepages/oxford_hip_score.html

Case 22

TIMEPOINT 1

Mr Walkins is a busy self-made entrepreneur. He developed diabetes 2 years ago and felt it must have been down to a combination of genetic and lifestyle factors. His father and uncle had diabetes. He knew he was overweight for some years, and was frustrated at himself for not being more particular about optimal diet and exercise during intense time periods developing his business. He can find a record that he had a BMI of 34 around 6 years ago, and it had not really changed since.

He was told that he was most likely to have type 2 diabetes – although he couldn't be sure as it had also been suggested that he might have a genetic type with just one gene responsible. Another friend reassured him that type 2 diabetes was 'mild', and he ignored the GP practice inviting him for 'foot checks' and invitations for eye screening as he thought that those were not his priority until he'd had the condition for at least 5 years. He had little detail in his past medical history apart from a previous inner ear infection leading to left-sided hearing loss.

His awareness that damage to nerves and other organs could occur in diabetes was balanced by the sense that he felt it unlikely that they would happen to him, although he had recently noticed a 'cotton wool' sensation on the soles of his feet. Three days earlier, he had remembered stepping on a rusty old nail, had fallen asleep early excessively tired and had just not inspected the soles of his feet since. He now has noticed a large, deep blistering lesion on the sole of his right foot. He goes and sees his GP as an emergency that morning, and the GP sends him to an ambulatory care medical unit the same day.

His observations are:

Respiratory rate: 17/min
Oxygen saturations: 96% on room air
Temperature: 37.8°C
Blood pressure: 160/88 mmHg
Heart rate: 90 bpm

Mr Walkins arrives at ambulatory care and is found to have a large 4×4 cm lesion to the medial aspect of the right foot.

The capillary blood glucose is 19.7 mmol/L. Mr Walkins has initial blood tests done, the results of which are shown below.

Venous blood results

Haemoglobin	130 g/L
White cell count	17 × 10⁹/L
Platelets	497 × 10⁹/L
CRP	214 mg/L

Intravenous antibiotics, a subcutaneous insulin regime, prophylactic dalteparin and medication appropriate for lipid management are all initiated, and admission to a short-stay unit is arranged. That night, the duty doctor is asked to review Mr Walkins due to ongoing fever, but incidentally notices a drug error that the dalteparin dose given earlier that day had been double the correct dose, due to incorrect weight and renal function dose estimation. That duty doctor completes an incident form to report the error.

Why is completing an incident form an important thing to do?

The completion of an incident form is a component of a multi-faceted approach to improve patient safety in healthcare settings. High-reporting organisations have been shown to learn more from those episodes, alongside 'near misses'. The data found within incident reports can be used to enable changes that may prevent events taking place in a similar way in the future.

TIMEPOINT ⏱ 2

Forty-eight hours later, the ward doctor managing Mr Walkins has seen steady improvement of the foot, stable glycaemia on the ward and detailed review by the hospital diabetic foot team. That morning, his observations show:

Respiratory rate: 18/min
Oxygen saturations: 96% on room air
Temperature: 37.7°C
Blood pressure: 130/72 mmHg
Heart rate: 81 bpm

Mr Walkins' current bloods show:

Venous blood results

Haemoglobin	136 g/L
White cell count	16×10^9/L
Platelets	74×10^9/L
CRP	205 mg/L

The diabetic foot team talks in detail as to whether the severity of the situation requires surgery, but it is felt preferable that medical treatment is continued.

Mr Walkins is very relieved because he remembers an uncle of his having foot surgery for a similar situation but being hugely shocked to discover that the lesion did not turn out to be what was expected when analysed histologically.

> Never assume that a diabetic foot ulcer on visual inspection is just that, especially if there are atypical features; always check the histology when excision of any kind takes place as primary or secondary cutaneous malignancy is an important differential.

When checking the day's blood results, the ward doctor is startled to see Mr Walkins'

platelet count. He calls the on-call consultant haematologist who suggests stopping all dalteparin or any other forms of heparin and doing 'HIT' bloods.

What is HIT?

Heparin-induced thrombocytopenia (HIT) is most likely with unfractionated heparin but can happen with any form – including low molecular weight. The significant risk posed by the condition is the risk of thrombotic events – the mechanism of which is not fully understood – and the challenges of treating them.

There are several scoring systems for HIT, one of which is the 4 Ts Score:

- *Thrombocytopenia* – degree of platelet count reduction
- *Timing* of platelet count fall
- *Thrombotic* events or similar
- *Thrombocytopenia* – absence of other causes for it

TIMEPOINT ⏱ 3

Twenty-four hours later, the ward-based resident doctor continues to be very concerned about the thrombocytopenia and worries that maybe it wasn't HIT but could be down to sepsis.

The following results are obtained:

Venous blood results

Haemoglobin	128 g/L
White cell count	13×10^9/L
Platelets	89×10^9/L
CRP	183 mg/L

Another phone conversation with a haematologist takes place, which in essence concludes with the haematologist advising that they still feel HIT is the most likely cause, and to continue managing the situation as per local HIT guidelines.

Why is HIT important?

It is significant as it can cause morbidity and mortality in severe forms and brings clinically challenging issues in order to resolve it without major sequelae. There are 2 major types – Type 1 and Type 2, Type 2 being more serious – and it takes place when a person treated with heparin develops a drug-related fall in platelet count. The risk that follows is unpredictable platelet-dense thrombotic events. It is associated with arterial thrombosis, adrenal failure, skin necrosis and limb gangrene.

Why is HIT difficult to diagnose?

Heparin is a very commonly prescribed medication, and thrombocytopenia can occur for many reasons. Therefore, a patient using heparin may have thrombocytopenia without it being 'heparin-induced' thrombocytopenia. To diagnose HIT, it is necessary to have a significant fall in platelets with timing consistent with heparin exposure, as well as thrombotic sequelae, with no other obvious cause of thrombocytopenia.

What is the treatment of HIT?

Treating HIT requires the discontinuation of heparin. In addition, there are possible treatment options in the form of a variety of pharmacological agents.

A non-heparin anticoagulant such as danaparoid or argatroban–warfarin can be considered, depending on thrombotic risk.

Expert senior haematological advice should be sought in all suspected cases of HIT.

TIMEPOINT ⏱ 4

At day 9 of admission, the blood tests for full blood count show normal results; thus the decision is that the heparin-induced thrombocytopenia has resolved. The following are results from that day:

Venous blood results

Haemoglobin	131 g/L
White cell count	10×10^9/L
Platelets	154×10^9/L
CRP	96 mg/L

The plans for discharging Mr Walkins are therefore made and recommendations made to aim to try and avoid being prescribed heparin in the future.

Later that day whilst waiting in the discharge lounge, Mr Walkins wonders whether he is more susceptible to deafness due to his diabetes. He does some research on his phone and finds out about other possible links between diabetes and hearing loss, and wonders if he might have a genetic condition.

There are two frequently encountered genetic conditions that directly combine diabetes and deafness: diabetes insipidus, diabetes mellitus, optic atrophy and deafness (DiDMOAD) and maternally inherited diabetes and deafness (MIDD). A pair of medical students who saw Mr Walkins throughout his stay go to visit him one more time prior to discharge. As they walk away from him, he mentions to them his thoughts about the genetic basis of disease and they leave discussing the relevant genetic conditions that they are aware of.

What are some of the patterns of high-penetrance inherited diseases?

In many clinical scenarios, potently inherited diseases have a particular pattern of transmission; major highly penetrant genetic conditions include:

Chromosomal conditions
- Trisomy 21 – Down syndrome
- XO – Turner syndrome
- XXY – Klinefelter syndrome

Autosomal-dominant conditions
- Multiple endocrine neoplasia (MEN)
- Familial hypercholesterolaemia
- Myotonic dystrophy
- Huntington disease
- Neurofibromatosis
- Polycystic kidney disease

Autosomal-recessive conditions
- Inborn errors of metabolism
- Alpha 1 antitrypsin deficiency
- Cystic fibrosis
- Sickle cell disease
- Tay–Sachs disease

X-linked recessive conditions
- Colour blindness
- Haemophilia
- Duchenne muscular dystrophy

Mitochondrial conditions
- Leber's hereditary optic neuropathy
- Kearns–Sayre syndrome

Case 23

TIMEPOINT ⏱ 1

Mr Davis is a 27-year-old banker who attends his GP because he is feeling tired all the time. He used to love working out at the gym, and would go at least every other day, but he has not been for the last couple of months because he has simply felt too exhausted by the time he gets home from work. Despite not going to the gym he has been losing weight, which he has assumed is because he has become very prone to diarrhoea over the last few months. He has noticed that even when he is not having diarrhoea, his stools have been particularly pale, smelly and difficult to flush which he has thought is strange. He has never seen any blood in his stool. He generally eats a healthy, varied and well-balanced diet to which he has not made any changes lately. No one in his family has ever had anything similar.

He has a background of type 1 diabetes mellitus for which he has an insulin pump. He also has a history of recurrent sinusitis and hay fever for which he uses saline and steroid nasal sprays as required. He does not take any other regular medications. He is allergic to peanuts but not to any medications that he is aware of. He is a teetotalling non-smoker. He lives with his girlfriend and their 3-year-old son.

His observations are:

Respiratory rate: 12/min
Oxygen saturations: 99% on room air
Temperature: 36.5°C
Blood pressure: 112/74 mmHg
Heart rate: 52 bpm

On examination he appears comfortable at rest. He is slim but not cachectic. There is obvious clubbing present. He appears slightly pale with conjunctival pallor. There is evidence of angular stomatitis around his mouth, and aphthous ulcers are noted on the mucous membranes. His abdomen is soft and non-tender with no palpable masses or organomegaly. PR examination is normal.

What are the causes of diarrhoea in adults?

- Gastrointestinal
  - Irritable bowel syndrome
  - Inflammatory bowel disease
  - Diverticular disease
  - Coeliac disease
  - Cancer of the GI tract
  - Overflow diarrhoea secondary to constipation
- Infectious
  - Bacterial, e.g. *Campylobacter jejuni*, *Clostridium difficile, Escherichia coli, Salmonella* spp., *Shigella* spp.
  - Viral, e.g. adenovirus, norovirus, rotavirus
  - Parasites, e.g. cryptosporidium, entamoeba, giardia
- Non-gastrointestinal infections, e.g. appendicitis
- Traveller's diarrhoea
- Drug-induced, e.g. secondary to laxatives, alcohol, caffeine, antibiotics, NSAIDs, proton-pump inhibitors, metformin, SSRIs, statins
- Food allergy or intolerance
- Bile salt malabsorption
- Pancreatic insufficiency secondary to pancreatitis, pancreatic cancer, cystic fibrosis
- Hyperthyroidism
- Radiation enteritis
- Stress/anxiety

The GP is unsure if this is either irritable bowel syndrome, inflammatory bowel disease or coeliac disease. He decides to send some blood tests to help him decide. The GP requests a number of

DOI: 10.1201/9781351257725-23

Table 23.1 Venous blood results

White cell count	7.4×10^9/L	Corrected calcium	2.31 mmol/L
Haemoglobin	118 g/L	CRP	12 mg/L
Platelets	237×10^9/L	Albumin	32 g/L
MCV	84 fL	Bilirubin	8 µmol/L
ESR	4 mm/hr	Alkaline phosphatase	58 U/L
Sodium	139 mmol/L	Alanine aminotransferase	27 U/L
Potassium	4.0 mmol/L	B12	259 ng/L
Urea	4.2 mmol/L	Folate	1.2 ng/mL
Creatinine	77 µmol/L	Ferritin	7 µg/L
Free T4	16.9 pmol/L	Tissue transglutaminase (IgA-TG2)	Negative
TSH	3.2 mU/L		

the blood tests and sends Mr Davis to the phlebotomist next door with the request forms. He promises to phone with the results. Until then, he suggests that Mr Davis keep a food diary in order to see if there is any pattern to his symptoms.

Later that evening, the GP is reviewing the blood test results (Table 23.1).

He sees that the tissue transglutaminase is negative, so he calls Mr Davis to advise him that he does not have coeliac disease. He thinks that inflammatory bowel disease is unlikely because there is no evidence of inflammation. He explains that he probably has irritable bowel syndrome and should try using the food diary to see which foods are triggering him. He also tells Mr Davis that he is quite anaemic which is probably contributing to him feeling tired all the time. He writes a prescription for folate and iron supplements and asks Mr Davis to pick them up from the front desk. He asks Mr Davis to book an appointment to see him again in 3 weeks' time with his food diary.

What are the symptoms of iron and B12 deficiencies, and how should they be managed?

See Table 23.2.

Management
- What is the underlying cause? This must be considered in addition to providing treatment. For example, iron-deficiency anaemia may be normal in a menstruating woman, but would be abnormal in a middle-aged man. If the patient has clear symptoms of

malabsorption, this is likely to explain an anaemia, but what is the underlying cause of the malabsorption? Consider whether further investigations are indicated, including endoscopy
- Iron deficiency can be treated with oral iron supplements. Iron can be given intravenously if the patient is unable to tolerate or does not take the oral supplements. Intravenous iron may also be useful in patients with malabsorption
- B12 deficiency is treated with IM hydroxocobalamin
- A dietician referral may be helpful in both cases

Key point

B12 must be replaced before folate (if folate is also deficient) to prevent the development or worsening of subacute combined degeneration of the cord.

TIMEPOINT ⏱ 2

Three weeks later, Mr Davis returns to the surgery with his food diary and sees a different GP. His symptoms have not improved since his last visit. They review the food diary together and notice that his bowels tend to be affected more on days when he has had sandwiches or pasta for lunch. On days when he has rice-based

Table 23.2 Symptoms of iron and B12 deficiency

	Iron-deficiency anaemia	Both	B12-deficiency anaemia
Causes	Blood loss	Poor diet Malabsorption	Pernicious anaemia
Symptoms and signs	Koilonychia Post-cricoid webs (Plummer–Vinson syndrome)	Glossitis Angular stomatitis Pallor of skin and conjunctiva Fatigue Shortness of breath on exertion Palpitations	Depression Psychosis Dementia Peripheral neuropathy Subacute combined degeneration of the cord
Blood film	Hypochromic microcytic erythrocytes with poikilocytosis and anisocytosis		Macrocytic with megaloblasts and hypersegmented polymorphs

dishes or baked potatoes, he doesn't seem to be as symptomatic.

The GP comments that Mr Davis' symptoms seem to flare when he eats gluten-containing products, which would be suggestive of coeliac disease. Mr Davis says that he agrees, but the last GP he saw told him that he didn't have coeliac disease. The GP says that given how typical his symptoms have been, he would like Mr Davis to do another blood test just to double check. Mr Davis agrees to this.

The GP resends a sample for tissue transglutaminase and requests an immunoglobulin panel (Table 23.3).

Reviewing the results later in the evening, the GP realises that the diagnosis of coeliac disease was initially missed as Mr Davis has selective IgA deficiency. He phones Mr Davis to explain what has happened and apologise for the fact that his diagnosis has been delayed. He tells Mr Davis that he will refer him to a gastroenterologist urgently. In the meantime he should continue to eat gluten-containing foods until he has a biopsy to confirm the diagnosis. He also refers Mr Davis to a clinical immunologist for their specialist input.

What are the key features of selective IgA deficiency?

- Background
  - It is the most common type of primary immunodeficiency, affecting around 1 in 500–600 people
  - Patients have a tendency towards
    - Allergy and atopy (food allergies, allergic rhinitis, asthma, eczema)
    - Autoimmunity (type 1 diabetes mellitus, vitiligo, rheumatoid arthritis, Grave's disease, SLE, myasthenia gravis)
    - Recurrent infections (usually sinus, respiratory and ear)
  - Both coeliac disease and inflammatory bowel disease are more common in IgA-deficient patients
  - There is also evidence that they are at increased risk of cancers, especially those of the GI tract
  - The majority are asymptomatic and many cases are discovered incidentally
- Management
  - Patients may be screened for allergic and autoimmune diseases if they have relevant symptoms

Table 23.3 Immunoglobulin test results

Test	Result	Reference range
IgA-TG2	Negative	
IgG-TG2	Positive	
IgG	12.4 g/L	6.0–16.0 g/L
IgA	0.1 g/L	0.8–4.5 g/L
IgM	1.5 g/L	0.5–2.0 g/L

- In patients with severe disease, live vaccines should be avoided and prophylactic antibiotics should be considered
- Patients may benefit from intravenous or subcutaneous immunoglobulin (although there is a risk of anaphylaxis from anti-IgA antibodies)
- There is also a rare risk of blood transfusion reactions due to presence of anti-IgA antibodies

What are other important causes of primary and secondary immunodeficiency?

- Primary
  - Combined variable immunodeficiency – variable defects in immunoglobulins and/or T-cells, depending on precise mutations
  - X-linked (Bruton's) agammaglobulinaemia – mutations blocking B-cell maturation, so very low levels of immunoglobulin produced
  - DiGeorge syndrome – absent or hypoplastic thymus leading to T-cell deficiencies
  - Hyper IgM syndrome – patients have abnormal T-cells so are unable to undergo immunoglobulin isotype switching. As a result, IgM levels are normal or high, but levels of IgG, IgA and IgE are low
  - Severe combined immunodeficiency – mutation leading to abnormal interleukin receptors prevents maturation of all aspects of the immune system. This results in low levels of T-cells, low levels of NK cells and normal numbers of non-functional B-cells
- Secondary
  - Cytotoxic drugs or immunosuppressive drugs, including chemotherapy, disease-modifying anti-rheumatic drugs (DMARDs), anti-rejection drugs given after organ transplantation, steroids
  - Disorders of the bone marrow including myeloma, myelodysplasia, leukaemia and lymphoma
  - Splenectomy

- Chronic illness including diabetes mellitus, cirrhosis, nephrotic syndromes
- Malnutrition
- Burns
- HIV (AIDS)

How can patients be tested for coeliac disease if they are known to be IgA-deficient?

IgG tissue transglutaminase (IgG-TG2) antibodies or IgG deamidated antigliadin (IgG-DGP) antibodies may be tested. Another option if there is reasonable confidence in the diagnosis is to send the patient for biopsy immediately without serological testing.

TIMEPOINT 3

Two weeks later, Mr Davis attends the hospital for an oesophagogastroduodenoscopy (OGD) and biopsy.

What are the diagnostic and therapeutic indications for OGD?

- Diagnostic
  - Biopsy for tissue diagnosis of coeliac disease or cancer
  - Dysphagia – achalasia, oesophageal cancer
  - Persistent dyspepsia/reflux despite a trial of therapy or dyspepsia with red flags – oesophageal or gastric cancer, peptic ulcer, hiatus hernia, achalasia
  - Melena, haematemesis, unexplained iron deficiency anaemia or suspicion of bleeding with negative colonoscopy – upper GI bleeding, underlying cancer
  - Investigation of radiologically confirmed oesophageal stricture
  - Surveillance of varices and in Barrett's oesophagus
- Therapeutic
  - Injection or argon plasma coagulation of bleeding ulcers or other lesions
  - Variceal banding or sclerotherapy
  - Removal of foreign body

- Dilatation or stenting of strictures
- Polypectomy
- PEG tube insertion

Mr Davis is sedated and undergoes a successful OGD. Five biopsy specimens are obtained and sent to the laboratory for analysis.

What are the key clinical features of coeliac disease on biopsy?

- Villous atrophy
- Crypt hyperplasia
- Increased intraepithelial T lymphocytes (>30 IEL/100 enterocytes)
- Flattening of enterocytes

TIMEPOINT  4

Six weeks later, Mr Davis attends his GP again for a follow-up after his biopsy. He has already seen the gastroenterologist, who has told him that his biopsies confirm coeliac disease. He has been seen by a dietician who has helped him to make his diet gluten-free. He tells the GP that he is getting on well and his symptoms have already improved significantly.

The gastroenterologist has suggested that Mr Davis do some reading about coeliac disease so that he feels more empowered. He has started to read but still has some questions for the GP. Mr Davis has read that having coeliac disease means that he is at an increased risk of having certain other diseases, but he is not sure which.

Which diseases are known to be associated with coeliac disease?

Coeliac disease is an autoimmune condition, and therefore patients are at increased risk of having another autoimmune disease. There are also various other conditions with no autoimmune component which seem to be associated with coeliac disease.

- Autoimmune disorders
  - Dermatitis herpetiformis
  - Type 1 diabetes mellitus
  - Autoimmune thyroid disease (more commonly hypothyroidism than hyperthyroidism)
  - Autoimmune hepatitis
  - Primary biliary cirrhosis
- Osteoporosis – may develop as a complication of undiagnosed or poorly managed coeliac disease due to calcium malabsorption
- Lactose intolerance
- Selective IgA deficiency
- Lymphoma and cancers of the GI tract
- Eosinophilic oesophagitis
- Inflammatory bowel disease
- Infertility or subfertility in both males and females

Mr Davis thanks the GP for answering his question. He has also been wondering if he is likely to develop food allergies now that he has coeliac disease. He would like to know what symptoms he should look out for, and how a food allergy can be investigated if it is suspected.

What questions should be asked in a food allergy history?

- When did the symptoms start?
- What symptoms are occurring?
- Which food(s) seems to trigger symptoms? How much food is needed to trigger a reaction?
- How quickly do symptoms occur after eating the food? Do the symptoms always occur after eating the food? How long do the symptoms last?
- Is there any personal or family history of allergy or atopy?

Which symptoms, if experienced after eating a trigger food, may be suggestive of a food allergy?

- Gastrointestinal symptoms
  - Reflux
  - Diarrhoea +/– blood +/– mucus
  - Constipation
  - Abdominal pain
  - Nausea and vomiting

- Dermatological and atopic symptoms
  - Eczema
  - Urticaria
  - Pruritus
  - Sneezing
  - Rhinorrhoea
  - Conjunctivitis
  - Wheeze
  - Shortness of breath
- Miscellaneous
  - Signs of anaphylaxis such as angio-oedema, stridor or cardiorespiratory compromise
  - Fatigue
  - Tailing growth
  - Food avoidance

How can a suspected food allergy be tested?

- Elimination diet
  - The suspected allergen is removed from the diet
  - If symptoms improve then the food should be reintroduced
  - If symptoms return after reintroduction this is suggestive of allergy
  - Should be supervised by a dietician
- Skin prick testing
  - A drop of food is placed on the forearm, then a needle is used to make a tiny break in the skin underneath the allergen
  - Development of a weal at the site is suggestive of allergy
  - May rarely cause anaphylaxis
- Blood testing
  - Assays may be used to test for serum allergen-specific IgE
  - No risk of anaphylaxis
- Challenge testing
  - Patient given increasing doses of suspected allergen orally until a reaction is provoked
  - Potentially high risk of anaphylaxis so should always be performed where resuscitation facilities are available

Case 24

TIMEPOINT 1

Mr Thine is a 52-year-old highly respected and introverted hospital porter who has become stressed recently due to colleague absence. From a health viewpoint, he'd been an infrequent GP attender and felt unsure what to do when previously a check-up had included mention of raised weight and blood pressure. He attended a celebratory ceremony for his 30 years' service to the NHS. He did not like the excessive attention this brought, and he found the experience both oddly uplifting but a bit overwhelming. He went to sleep feeling unsettled that night, and he began to feel very unwell before his shift the very next morning and called an ambulance at 0646 as he was suffering with new onset chest pains.

He arrives looking pale and sweaty and feels uneasy to be a patient at his workplace.

Observations and an ECG had been carried out by the paramedics en route. His observations showed:

Respiratory rate: 24/min
Oxygen saturations: 96% on room air
Temperature: 37°C
Blood pressure: 167/97 mmHg
Heart rate: 97 bpm

His height and weight were also checked and his BMI calculated. His height was 1.8 m, weight 112 kg and BMI 34.6.

The 12 lead ECG showed ST depression in the inferior leads (II, III and AVF).

The emergency department team see Mr Thine and make an initial assessment. It is clear the duty cardiologist should be involved soon, but beforehand a history, examination and relevant investigations are arranged. The history reveals this as a new episode of cardiac-sounding chest pain. He had previously wondered about 'taking an aspirin a day' but it was not recommended as the only positive risk factors were an ex-smoker status of 20 pack-years and a positive family history. Examination is unremarkable. Routine blood tests, including troponin level, a repeat ECG and chest X-ray are all ordered.

The results show a raised high-sensitivity troponin I level of 249 ng/L, and a cholesterol level of 6.3 mmol/L.

What are the risk factors for ischemic coronary artery disease?

The major risk factors can be categorised into modifiable and non-modifiable (Table 24.1).

TIMEPOINT 2

The duty cardiology doctor starts NSTEMI treatment using an NSTEMI treatment in hospital pathway.

This includes:

- Fondaparinux: 2.5 mg SC OD
- Aspirin: 300 mg stat then 75 mg OD
- Clopidogrel: 300 mg stat then 75 mg OD
- Bisoprolol: titrated upwards
- Ramipril: titrated upwards
- Atorvastatin: 80 mg ON

Mr Thine is admitted to the acute cardiac unit on continuous telemetry ECG monitoring.

What is fondaparinux?

Fondaparinux sodium is an anticoagulant, somewhat similar to low-molecular-weight heparins, and is a synthetic pentasaccharide that inhibits activated factor X.

DOI: 10.1201/9781351257725-24

Table 24.1 Risk factors for ischaemic coronary artery disease

Modifiable	Non-modifiable
• Smoking	• Increasing age
• Dyslipidaemia	• Family history
• Obesity	• Genetic factors affecting lipids
• Diabetes	• Genetic impact of conditions such as homocystinaemia
• Hypertension	
• Psychosocial stress	

TIMEPOINT ⏲ 3

The following morning, the attending consultant cardiologist sees Mr Thine on the acute cardiac ward round. He goes through the significance of the positive troponin and ECG changes. He assesses the sequence of events and has a discussion with Mr Thine concluding in a decision to do an inpatient angiogram.

What is coronary angiography?

A coronary angiogram is a central investigation for coronary heart disease. It is both diagnostic and potentially therapeutic. It helps with the diagnostic process by ascertaining whether or not coronary vasospasm or any form of local arterial dissection is present. It also localises lesions of tight coronary artery stenosis. It is performed by a trained cardiologist via arterial puncture of the radial (or femoral artery), and radio-opaque contrast demonstrates the findings.

The angiogram reveals two-vessel stenosis, in the right coronary artery (RCA) and left anterior descending (LAD) artery; both are stented. Mr Thine makes a good recovery in hospital and is informed of the angiogram and stenting outcome. Prior to discharge, Mr Thine has a further ward review by the consultant cardiologist, alongside the rest of the cardiac medical nursing team and the cardiac rehabilitation nurse.

Advice from the cardiac rehabilitation nurse includes a range of recommendations, and she sets up an onward programme of group meetings. Topics discussed and included in the written leaflets provided include:

● Diet – particularly in relation to cholesterol
● Exercise – especially when to commence and appropriate levels of intensity
● Employment advice
● Driving advice
   ● In the UK, the Driver and Vehicle Licensing Agency issues guidance in relation to this on its website; in general, driving may resume 1 week after ACS if treated by successful coronary intervention (PCI) and 4 weeks after if not – precise details can be obtained via the DVLA

The pharmacist goes through all the discharging medications, including indications, contraindications and the overall rationale. Mr Thine is surprised to see so many tablets and did not know that patients are generally discharged taking a statin following any acute coronary syndrome. He asks for an information sheet about 'statins' which is entitled 'Hyperlipidaemia'.

Hyperlipidaemia

Hyperlipidaemia can be inherited or acquired – it is a very common key risk factor for all cardiovascular disease. Certain inherited aspects are potent and can accelerate the risk of coronary events; an important one is familial hypercholesterolaemia (FH). It is relevant to note that FH is usually transmitted in an autosomal-dominant fashion; other genetic patterns include it being polygenic or recessive.

The condition of hyperlipidaemia is linked with a variety of dietary factors, such as inactivity, obesity and alcohol intake, alongside various medical conditions such as nephrotic syndrome.

Managing hyperlipidaemia partly depends on the 10-year probability of a future cardiovascular event; previous cardiovascular events both for the individual and relatives; early response to medication; ethnicity; and patient preference. In addition, the presence of diabetes has an important influence.

Clinical signs suggestive of dyslipidaemia include tendon xanthomata and xanthelasma (a yellowish deposit of cholesterol on or around the eyelids).

Options for treatment start with diet and lifestyle optimisation, but medication is often recommended, and NICE UK guidelines have a threshold of 10-year risk (there are online calculators available) to estimate the need for treatment.

Drug treatment most commonly involves HMGCoA reductase inhibitors commonly known as 'statins'; there are several available but atorvastatin and simvastatin are most usually prescribed. Trial evidence for the use of a statin is extensive and has many years of outcome data that are generally favourable. A few patients experience statin side effects, notably muscle pain/raised CK.

An alternative lipid-lowering drug is ezetimibe, which is permitted to be used both instead of (such as following adverse reactions) or in combination with a statin.

Alternatively, some patients are prescribed a fibrate, e.g. bezafibrate.

Much more recently a range of targeted therapies, particularly used in genetic forms of diabetes, have become available, and they include alirocumab, evolocumab, lomitapide and inclisiran. Very carefully designed trials are beginning to see the potential for positive effects of these agents in a broader range of indications, and therefore it is likely they will become more extensively considered over time.

TIMEPOINT ⏱ 4

Two days later, after Mr Thine was discharged, he was told to return for a one-stop follow-up clinic. This includes a further meeting with a cardiac rehabilitation nurse and an echocardiogram. A professional cardiology multidisciplinary team (MDT) meets around lunchtime; resulting in Mr Thine being given the MDT outcome and future plans via consultation with a cardiac specialist nurse later that day.

The cardiology imaging MDT meeting examined evidence including angiogram analysis and the echocardiogram.

The angiogram showed:

76% stenosis of both the right coronary and left mainstem; both have been stented.

The echocardiogram showed:

Minor level of wall motion abnormality of left ventricle; EF estimated at 50%; AV/MV/TV/PV all normal; a suggestion of an atrial septal defect (ASD), which was directly followed by a bubble echo.

The bubble echo showed:

A clearly visualised ASD.

Mr Thine is informed of all these results and the MDT outcome, which was to reassure him that the left ventricular function was quite well-preserved and to set up plans to treat the ASD.

What are the key issues in the management of ASD in adulthood?

There are two categories of atrial septal defect commonly described: ostium primum and ostium secundum defects. In general, an ASD can be found incidentally or via investigation for dysrhythmias, atrial fibrillation or the finding of a pulmonary/tricuspid murmur.

There has been much debate as to when and whether to treat an ASD and other blood flow disorders. The main concern is 'paradoxical emboli'.

This condition results from an embolus of a deep vein thrombosis that, rather than entering the pulmonary circulation causing a pulmonary embolus, crosses the ASD and enters the systemic circulation causing either an ischaemic stroke or other arterial embolic event.

If the decision to treat the ASD is made, options include surgical closure or a transcatheter insertion of a helical/double umbrella device that straddles the defect and creates closure.

FURTHER READING

1. https://www.gov.uk/guidance/cardiovascular-disorders-assessing-fitness-to-drive

Case 25

TIMEPOINT 1

Mrs Wilks is a 65-year-old seamstress who arranged a routine GP appointment where her general health, lifestyle and alcohol intake were reviewed.

She had a past medical history of osteoarthritis and mild dyslipidaemia, for which not enough risk was felt to be present to require lipid-lowering treatment. She lives alone, takes no medication, has no allergies, smokes 4–5 cigarettes a day – for around 30 years – and admits to drinking around a bottle of wine every few days.

At the scheduled visit to her GP surgery she described intermittent palpitations for 3 months. Clinical examination reveals an irregularly irregular pulse. The GP arranges for an ECG, which shows atrial fibrillation (AF).

What three core treatment considerations are made in a patient with AF?

1. Rate control
2. Rhythm control
3. Anticoagulation

The GP decides that immediate consideration of rate control and anticoagulation is needed, but rhythm control/alteration is not immediately necessary, but would be a consideration in future. Bisoprolol is commenced for rate control. Anticoagulation is used in AF to reduce stroke risk and requires detailed consideration. The standard method is to use the CHA_2DS_2-VASc and HASBLED scores to determine whether to start anticoagulation or not, e.g., a CHA_2DS_2-VASc score of 2 or more, along with a low HASBLED score, would suggest it is appropriate to start anticoagulation. Mrs Wilks has full capacity to decide, and in the end declines any anticoagulant, i.e. not warfarin or a direct oral anticoagulant (DOAC). The GP recorded that he had quite clearly encouraged her to take a DOAC based on a CHA_2DS_2-VASc and HASBLED score.

What are the features of the CHA_2DS_2-VASc/HASBLED scoring system?

See Tables 25.1 and 25.2.

TIMEPOINT 2

Eight days later, Mrs Wilks is in a local cafe, when she falls off a stool. Mrs Wilks appears to have a drooping left side of the face and possibly floppy left arm. An ambulance is called straight away. She arrives at the hospital 50 minutes after the onset of symptoms.

On arrival, her observations are:

Respiratory rate: 19/min
Oxygen saturations: 99% on room air
Temperature: 37.2°C
Blood pressure: 178/114 mmHg
Heart rate: 89 bpm

Her GCS is 14/15 (disorientated).

Examination reveals an irregularly irregular pulse.

Neurologically, there is left-sided weakness of the face, arm and leg. Mrs Wilks' facial movements seem to show sparing of the forehead.

The stroke team is immediately consulted.

A CT head is performed minutes after arrival in the ED, showing no haemorrhage and possible initial features of left cerebral infarct.

The local stroke intervention protocol is used. Fortunately, Mrs Wilks is at a hospital with 24/7 access to thrombolysis decisions, although other thrombectomy treatments are only available at a tertiary referral centre. As thrombolysis criteria are met, intravenous thrombolytic therapy is given.

DOI: 10.1201/9781351257725-25

Table 25.1 CHA$_2$DS$_2$-VASc scoring system

CHA$_2$DS$_2$-VASc risk factors	
Congestive heart failure	1
Hypertension	1
Age ≥75	2
Age 65–74	1
Diabetes mellitus	1
Stroke/TIA/thrombo-embolism	2
Vascular disease	1
Sex female	1

Table 25.2 HASBLED scoring system

HASBLED clinical characteristics	
Hypertension	1
Abnormal liver function	1
Abnormal renal function	1
Stroke	1
Bleeding	1
Labile INRs	1
Elderly (age >65)	1
Drugs	1
Alcohol	1

What vascular interventions have been developed in acute ischemic stroke?

The last two decades have seen rapid advances in the options for improving outcomes in ischaemic stroke based on a 'time-is-brain' concept. In selected cases, pro-active interventions aimed at improved blood flow at and around the area of infarction bring about greater functional capability, post-rehabilitation. Large numbers of clinical trials have incorporated methods such as intravenous thrombolytic therapy, intra-arterial techniques and/or thrombectomy. These interventions are delivered following the confirmation that the stroke is indeed ischaemic (using brain imaging such as CT and, at times, various other forms of MRI scans). Thrombectomy is most frequently currently performed if the occlusive location is the internal carotid or M1 or M2 segments of the middle cerebral artery (there are four segments in total; M1–M4). The time-windows for these interventions are crucial. The National Institute of Neurological Disorders and Stroke (NINDS) scoring system, amongst others, can determine the correct level of severity for intervention. Thrombolysis decisions and similar decisions can be made via telemedicine. Further advancements include 'stroke ambulances' in some areas which incorporate a CT scanner inside the vehicle; in addition, new mobile CT scanners will improve access to imaging urgently.

TIMEPOINT ⏱ 3

Three hours later, Mrs Wilks is now on the stroke ward. On a regular review the staff nurse notes concerning observations:

Respiratory rate: 16/min
Oxygen saturations: 98% on room air
Temperature: 37.3°C
Blood pressure: 168/112 mmHg
Heart rate: 61 bpm
GCS: 6/15

The nurse is concerned about these observations, especially given that Mrs Wilks looks unwell and her GCS has dropped to 6/15. She immediately calls the on-call doctor who books a repeat CT scan as they are concerned about the possibility of a post-thrombolytic haemorrhage. The CT scan confirms a haemorrhage.

Why is blood pressure monitoring so important in the acute management of stroke?

Hypertension is a major influencing feature for stroke and post-stroke; blood pressure changes can signify various issues. It is thought large rises or falls in blood pressure post-stroke can be detrimental to the recovery of the affected area of brain. In addition, blood pressure can change as a 'Cushing's reflex' – whereby bradycardia and hypertension can reflect raised intracranial pressure.

The repeat CT scan is seen and assessed by the local duty neurosurgical team, and the decision is made not to do neurosurgery.

What is the reason for calling neurosurgeons when an acute stroke patient's condition changes?

In the above case, any post-stroke haemorrhage, whether or not in the context of being post-thrombolysis, will require neurosurgical opinion as to whether urgent surgical evacuation of the haemorrhage is indicated. There is a further scenario, known as malignant middle cerebral artery (MCA) syndrome, where developing oedema around the site of a large MCA infarct has been shown to affect the prognosis, and hemicraniectomy can be performed in selected cases.

TIMEPOINT ⏱ 4

Four months later, Mrs Wilks is now at home after several months of rehabilitation at various locations. Mrs Wilks' husband, children and friends all provide help given that she is quite severely affected by unilateral hemiplegia and spends significant amounts of time in a wheelchair. The national Stroke Association charity has provided online, telephone and local support; the local GP and practice nurses have been both visiting and looking to ensure the optimal psychological wellbeing of everyone concerned. The family has found this support incredibly helpful and collectively they feel they have enough arrangements in place to manage well for the future.

Why is psychological wellbeing important after stroke?

The severity of impact of stroke, both the effects on the brain itself and the challenges assessing the patient's communication about how they feel, means a high percentage – thought to be 20–30% – of patients suffer depression post-stroke. Stroke charities and health care teams are now well-aware of this and aim for both early detection and intervention.

What is the overall prognostic risk factor strategy to prevent further events after a stroke?

This involves careful attention to the major risk factors, dependent on whether the stroke was an infarct or haemorrhage. Investigation into the underlying source of the stroke is important. Where relevant, carotid dopplers, heart rhythm assessment and echocardiography may all contribute. If an infarct, appropriate anti-platelet treatment is needed, and if the patient is in AF, anticoagulation (starting 2 weeks post-infarct) should be considered. Raised blood pressure should be actively managed, lipid-lowering medication used and glycaemia well-managed. Smoking cessation support should also be actively a part of the management plan.

FURTHER READING

1. Meredith G., Rudd A. *Postgrad Med J* 2019;95:271–278.

Case 26

Mr Read is a 39-year-old man who presents to the emergency department because he is worried about how swollen his stomach has become over the last week. He usually works doing the paper round for his local newsagent, but has been too exhausted and nauseous to go to work the last few days, and now his boss is threatening to fire him if he doesn't go back to work tomorrow. He called an ambulance because he was feeling terrible, and didn't know what else to do. He wonders if the fact that he is feeling so unwell might be connected to his stomach.

The emergency department doctor is unable to trace Mr Read's medical history as he is not registered with a GP. He denies having any medical problems, taking any regular medications or having any allergies. He says that he has never smoked 'because it killed my father', and that he can't afford to drink alcohol.

His observations are:

Respiratory rate: 27/min
Oxygen saturations: 88% on room air
Temperature: 37.8°C
Blood pressure: 102/74 mmHg
Heart rate: 108 bpm

From the end of the bed, he appears breathless with an obviously distended abdomen. He is warm and well perfused with a capillary refill time of less than 2 seconds. There is no clubbing seen. There is evidence of track marks and bruising on both arms, and his muscles appear generally wasted. Scleral jaundice is noted. On the chest, seven spider naevi are seen. Heart sounds are normal, and there is good air entry bilaterally with no added sounds. The abdomen is significantly distended but non-tender. There is evidence of shifting dullness on percussion. Bowel sounds are normal but quiet.

The emergency department doctor asks Mr Read about the track marks on his arms, and whether he has ever been an intravenous drug user. Mr Read admits that he mostly injects cocaine but will use heroin when he can get hold of it. The doctor asks whether he has ever shared any needles used for injection. Mr Read says that he used to, but stopped at least 10 years ago. The emergency department doctor thanks Mr Read for his honesty and asks the nurse to fetch the ultrasound machine whilst he reviews the blood tests which were sent from triage (Table 26.1).

The emergency department doctor is concerned about Mr Read's deranged LFTs and distended abdomen. He performs a bedside ultrasound which shows evidence of large-volume ascites.

Which differential diagnoses should be considered for a patient with ascites?

- Decompensated liver disease
- Budd–Chiari syndrome
- Nephrotic syndrome
- Heart failure
- Malignancy of the gastrointestinal tract or intra-abdominal metastasis
- Lymphoma
- Meigs' syndrome
- Connective tissue disease
- Malnutrition
- Protein losing enteropathy
- Ovarian hyperstimulation
- Pancreatitis
- Tuberculosis

In light of the large-volume ascites, the emergency department doctor hands over to the gastroenterology team who decide to place an ascitic drain and send a liver screen.

DOI: 10.1201/9781351257725-26

Table 26.1 Venous blood results

White cell count	14.3×10^9/L	Urea	7.2 mmol/L
Haemoglobin	128 g/L	Creatinine	84 µmol/L
Platelets	420×10^9/L	Albumin	29 g/L
MCV	99 fL	Bilirubin	59 µmol/L
Sodium	136 mmol/L	Alkaline phosphatase	124 U/L
Potassium	4.3 mmol/L	Alanine aminotransferase	375 U/L

What should ascitic fluid be tested for when a sample is taken?

Paired blood samples must be taken for serum albumin, glucose and amylase.

Separate samples should be obtained for cell count (and differential), microscopy and culture (including Gram staining), cytology and biochemistry (Table 26.2).

The serum ascitic albumin gradient (SAAG) is a useful calculation which provides a proxy measure of portal pressure. It may be calculated as follows:

$$SAAG = \text{serum albumin} - \text{ascitic fluid albumin}$$

An SAAG $\geq$1.1 g/dL (11 g/L) is highly suggestive of portal hypertension. It also suggests that the ascites is more likely to be a transudate.

An SAAG <1.1 g/dL (11 g/L) is suggestive of an exudate.

Table 26.2 Interpretation of ascitic fluid results

	Result	Possible diagnosis
Albumin	0.3–4 g/dL	Normal
	>4 g/dL	SPB Tuberculosis
Glucose	Similar to serum level	Normal
	Lower than serum level	Tuberculosis Malignancy
Amylase	Similar to serum level	Normal
	Greater than serum level	Pancreatitis
Colour	Clear/straw	Normal Cirrhosis
	Cloudy	SBP Pancreatitis
	Bloody	Malignancy
	Milky	Malignancy Lymphoma Tuberculosis
White cell count	<250/mm^3	Normal Cirrhosis
	>250/mm^3, mostly neutrophils	SBP
	>250/mm^3, mostly lymphocytes	Tuberculosis
Red cell count	None	Normal
	>1000/mm^3	Tuberculosis Malignancy
	>100,000/mm^3	Haemorrhage

What would be concerning about an ascitic neutrophil count above 250 cells/mm³?

- This would be diagnostic of spontaneous bacterial peritonitis (SBP)
- SBP is an important complication of ascites
- It usually occurs in patients with advanced cirrhosis
- This can be asymptomatic, or may present with fever, abdominal pain and confusion
- It is predominantly caused by *Enterococci* spp., *Streptococcus* spp., *Klebsiella* spp. and *Escherichia coli*
- It is usually treated empirically with a third-generation cephalosporin, and then according to ascitic culture results
- Antibiotic prophylaxis with a quinolone reduces risk of recurrence. Prophylaxis may also be appropriate in other high-risk groups
- Patients who have had an episode of SBP should be considered for liver transplantation given the high 2-year mortality (50%)

Placement of the ascitic drain goes well, and the gastroenterology doctors review Mr Read's liver screen (Table 26.3).

He also has imaging, including a normal chest X-ray and an ultrasound scan showing significant cirrhotic changes but no evidence of malignancy. Transient elastography (Fibroscan) gives a median liver stiffness of 32 kPa which is highly suggestive of cirrhosis.

The gastroenterology doctor explains to Mr Read that his ascites has been caused by severe liver cirrhosis secondary to chronic hepatitis C. It is likely that he contracted the hepatitis C from a contaminated needle when he was injecting drugs many years ago. The gastroenterology doctor refers Mr Read to a hepatologist to discuss starting antiviral treatment. He also arranges for him to attend counselling regarding his new diagnosis. Mr Read is advised to start a fluid- and salt-restricted diet and is started on furosemide and spironolactone to try and prevent the ascites from recurring. He makes a good recovery from the acute episode and is discharged 4 days later.

TIMEPOINT ⏱ 2

Four months later, Mr Read attends the emergency department saying that he has vomited up a small amount of very dark brown vomit today with some streaks of blood in. He has had worsening abdominal pain for the last 48 hours and feels generally unwell. He has also noticed that his stools are becoming increasingly dark and have a tar-like consistency. His chronic hepatitis C is now being managed by the hepatology team, who have started him on oral ribavirin daily and once weekly peginterferon alpha injections.

From the end of the bed, Mr Read appears pale.

His observations are:

Respiratory rate: 16/min
Oxygen saturations: 98% on room air

Table 26.3 Liver screen results

α1 antitrypsin	Normal	Hepatitis A (anti-HAV antibodies)	Negative
Alpha fetoprotein	Negative	Hepatitis B (surface antigen)	Negative
Anti-mitochondrial antibodies	Negative	Hepatitis B (anti-core antibodies)	Negative
Anti-nuclear antibodies	Negative	**Hepatitis C (anti-HCV antibodies)**	**POSITIVE**
Anti-smooth muscle antibodies	Negative	**Hepatitis C (viral RNA)**	**POSITIVE**
Caeruloplasmin	Normal	Hepatitis E (anti-HEV antibodies)	Negative
Copper	Normal	HIV	Negative
Cytomegalovirus IgG	Negative	INR	1.3
Epstein–Barr virus antibodies	Negative	Lipid profile	Normal
Ferritin	Raised	Free thyroxine (FT4)	17 pmol/L
Gamma glutamyl transferase	Normal	Thyroid-stimulating hormone	3.1 mU/L

Temperature: 37.7°C
Blood pressure: 107/66 mmHg
Heart rate: 88 bpm

The emergency department doctor starts to examine Mr Read. He is cool peripherally with a capillary refill time of 4 seconds. He is checking Mr Read's pulse manually when he has another episode of haematemesis, consisting of a large volume of fresh red blood. He asks a nurse to put out a peri-arrest call as he is now very worried about Mr Read.

More members of staff start to arrive for the peri-arrest call. The emergency department doctor asks one to bring the crash trolley and to start cannulating and taking bloods and one to fast bleep the on-call gastroenterologist while he assesses Mr Read again.

How should Mr Read be managed acutely?

Mr Read should be assessed and resuscitated using a DRABCDE scheme (Table 26.4).

Mr Read's observations during this assessment are:

Respiratory rate: 24/min
Oxygen saturations: 94% on room air
Temperature: 37.9°C
Blood pressure: 98/67 mmHg
Heart rate: 123 bpm

Table 26.4 DRABCDE management scheme

D – Danger	• Assess if there is danger before approaching the patient – spills, wires, etc.
R – Response	• Does the patient respond to verbal or painful stimulation? Assess GCS/AVPU
	• If no response, assess for signs of life. If no signs of life, call for help and commence BLS/ALS
A – Airway	• Look for any airway obstruction, e.g. vomit, blood
	• Listen for added airway sounds, e.g. stridor
	• If any concerns, call for help. Maintain airway using basic manoeuvres and adjuncts if needed
	• If patient can talk, airway is patent
B – Breathing	• Check respiratory rate and oxygen saturations
	• Look for movement of chest wall, cyanosis, accessory muscle use
	• Auscultate chest for wheeze or crepitations
	• Oxygen if signs of respiratory distress or confusion
	• Consider an ABG and chest X-ray
C – Circulation	• Check heart rate, blood pressure and JVP
	• Check capillary refill time – is the patient perfused peripherally?
	• Look for pallor and evidence of bleeding
	• 2x wide-bore cannulae
	• Bloods including FBC, U&E, LFT, coagulation screen
	• Crossmatch at least two units
	• IV fluid challenges initially, then give blood as soon as available
	• ECG and commence cardiac monitoring
	• Catheter insertion with urometer
D – Disability	• Reassess GCS/AVPU
	• Check blood glucose
E – Exposure and everything else	• Top-to-toe examination
	• Urgent endoscopy with band ligation or sclerotherapy to stem the bleeding
	• Start terlipressin
	• Start prophylactic antibiotics (ciprofloxacin)
	• Calculate Blatchford and Rockall scores

Table 26.5 Venous blood results

White cell count	12.4×10^9/L	Sodium	139 mmol/L
Haemoglobin	104 g/L	Potassium	5.1 mmol/L
Platelets	167×10^9/L	Urea	12.2 mmol/L
MCV	96 fL	Creatinine	118 µmol/L

His initial blood test results are given in Table 26.5.

The gastroenterologist on call arrives and starts to calculate Mr Read's Blatchford and pre-endoscopy Rockall scores.

How are Blatchford and Rockall scores calculated? What are Mr Read's scores?

The Blatchford score predicts the risk of a bleeding patient needing a transfusion, endoscopy or

Table 26.6 Blatchford score

Blatchford score marker	Value	Score
Urea (mmol/L)	6.5–7.9	2
	8.0–9.9	3
	10.0–24.9	**4**
	≥25	6
Haemoglobin – men (g/dL)	≥12–13	1
	10–11.9	**3**
	<10	6
Haemoglobin – women (g/dL)	≥10–12	1
	<10	6
Systolic blood pressure (mmHg)	100–109	1
	90–99	**2**
	<90	3
Pulse	≥100	**1**
Melena	-	**1**
Syncope	-	2
Hepatic disease	-	**2**
Cardiac failure	-	2

Table 26.7 Rockall pre-endoscopy score

Rockall pre-endoscopy score marker	Value	Score
Age (years)	60–79	1
	≥80	2
Shock	Tachycardia: Systolic blood pressure ≥100 AND pulse ≥100	1
	Hypotension: Systolic blood pressure <100	**2**
Comorbidities	Any comorbidity EXCEPT liver failure, renal failure or malignancy	2
	Liver failure, renal failure or malignancy	**3**

surgery. It is most useful when assessing patients in the emergency department who are being considered for hospital admission. A score is calculated between 0 and 23. Patients with a low score may be safe to manage as outpatients. A score of ≥6 is associated with a >50% risk of needing one of those interventions (Table 26.6).

Mr Read's Blatchford score would be 13.

The Rockall score is used to estimate mortality in patients with active upper gastrointestinal bleeding. There are two versions which can be calculated depending on whether the patient has had endoscopy yet or not. It is a well-validated score which is easy to use (Table 26.7).

Mr Read's pre-endoscopy Rockall score would therefore be 5, correlating with a 39.6% mortality risk prior to endoscopy. A score of 0 correlates with a 0.2% risk of mortality, increasing to 50% with a score of 7.

The post-endoscopy ('complete') score includes scoring for the diagnosis and stigmata of haemorrhage, and predicts both the mortality risk and the risk of rebleeding.

Mr Read is resuscitated with fluids and two units of blood and then taken directly to endoscopy where severe variceal bleeding is seen, so proceeds to urgent variceal banding. The procedure goes well and he is transferred to the gastroenterology ward later in the evening.

TIMEPOINT ⏱ 3

The following morning after the endoscopy, Mr Read's full blood count is repeated for review on the gastroenterology ward round (Table 26.8).

He has not had any further bleeding overnight. He reports that he is generally feeling better but feels dizzy every time he tries to stand up. The consultant says that he thinks Mr Read should have another two units of blood transfused and asks the junior doctor on the team to sort this out at the end of the ward round.

Table 26.8 **Venous blood results**

White cell count	13.6×10^9/L
Haemoglobin	76 g/L
Platelets	189×10^9/L
MCV	72 fL

What information should be included when consenting patients for a blood transfusion?

As with all forms of consent, patients should have the procedure explained to them in an appropriate level of detail, including the reason that it is required. They should be informed about the risks and benefits of the procedure, and also the alternative treatment options if they choose to decline the procedure. Written consent is not routinely required from the patient for blood transfusion, but there should be clear documentation in the notes that the patient has received a full explanation and verbally consented. Adults with capacity are always entitled to refuse a treatment, even life-saving ones, and even if the medical professional believes that decision to be unwise. If a patient does not have capacity, the decision should be made in the patient's best interests.

Example of consent for blood transfusion:

- Explanation of procedure
  - We would like to give you a blood transfusion because (clinical indication)
  - We hope that symptom X/Y/Z (e.g. shortness of breath, feeling dizzy or lightheaded) will improve with the transfusion
  - This will involve us taking a blood test to check your blood group
  - Once we know your blood group, we will give you (x number) units of blood
  - The blood is given through a drip in your arm. One unit usually takes around 3 hours to be given
  - While you are receiving the blood, we will monitor you more carefully to make sure that you aren't reacting badly to it
- Risks
  - There is a very small risk of having a reaction to the blood
  - We will monitor you carefully and if we think this is happening we will stop the transfusion immediately to make sure that you are safe
  - There is also a tiny risk of contracting an infection, however, all blood products

are now screened for infections to ensure that this doesn't happen, so this is now extremely rare

- Benefits
  - The transfusion should improve your blood count (haemoglobin level) which is important for your general health
  - The transfusion will help to replace the blood that you lost when you were bleeding/during the surgery
  - The benefit of the transfusion is that you should start to feel better/symptoms X/Y/Z should improve
- Alternatives
  - Alternatives may include iron tablets or iron transfusions
  - Iron tablets may be an option in patients keen to avoid a transfusion. However, they take a long time to work so may not be good if your blood count is already very low to the point where it is making you feel unwell. They can also cause constipation
  - Intravenous iron may be an option in some cases, but it is generally more effective to use a blood transfusion
- Gaining consent
  - Are you happy to go ahead with the transfusion?
  - Is there anything that is unclear that you would like me to explain again?
  - Do you have any questions?

What are the possible complications of blood transfusion?

- Acute haemolytic transfusion reaction
  - This occurs when the patient receives ABO-incompatible blood, or blood with another incompatible major antigen
  - Complement is activated leading to intravascular haemolysis, disseminated intravascular coagulation and shock
  - This is usually due to human error which is why transfusion-checking procedures are now so strict
  - Symptoms and signs include hypotension, nausea and vomiting, abdominal pain, chest pain, anxiety and fever

- If there are any concerns, the transfusion should be stopped immediately and the blood returned to the laboratory for retesting
- Repeat blood tests should be taken from the patient, including a full blood count, crossmatch, coagulation screen and any antibody testing advised by the blood bank
- Give intravenous fluids and oxygen. Monitor the patient's urine output. Consider early escalation to intensive care if hypotensive
- Alloimmunisation
  - Not an issue with the initial transfusion but may cause a problem if transfused at a later date
- Anaphylaxis and allergy
  - Occurs if the recipient has antibodies against components of the transfused blood products
  - If there is evidence of anaphylaxis, the transfusion should be stopped and the patient managed as per usual anaphylaxis protocol
  - If only evidence of pruritus and rash but systemically well, can usually be managed by slowing the transfusion and giving antihistamines
- Delayed haemolysis
  - Presents with jaundice, haemoglobinuria and fevers approximately 1 week post-transfusion
  - Patients have antibodies which may have been undetectable at crossmatching, but levels of which increase after transfusion causing destruction of the transfused cells
- Febrile reaction
  - This is a common reaction which is not dangerous (if mild fever is the only symptom)
  - Fever and rigors may occur if the recipient has antibodies against transfused white cells
  - Manage by slowing the transfusion and giving paracetamol
- Fluid overload

- Can occur if any fluid is transfused too quickly, or too great a volume is transfused
- Can result in pulmonary oedema, leading to respiratory distress and failure
- Patients known to be high risk (e.g. pre-existing heart failure) may require diuretic therapy concurrently with the transfusion
- Graft versus host disease
  - Caused by the recipient reacting to T-cells in the transfusion
  - Immunosuppressed patients are at risk
  - Can be prevented by using irradiated blood products
- Infection
  - Infection can occur due to contamination of the blood product
  - Blood-borne viruses (HIV, hepatitis B, hepatitis C) can also be transferred
  - Both are extremely rare but potentially very serious
  - Contamination occurs more commonly with platelets than red cells as red cells are stored at cooler temperatures
  - All blood products are now screened for viruses, and those with existing infection are not allowed to donate
  - Symptoms may be difficult to distinguish from an acute haemolytic reaction or allergic reaction – take blood cultures if concerned
- Iron overload
  - Patients at risk should receive desferrioxamine chelation
- Transfusion-related acute lung injury
  - This occurs when the donated blood contains antibodies against the leucocytes in the lungs of the recipient
  - Patients develop acute respiratory distress with shortness of breath, cough and hypoxia. They may also appear systemically unwell and febrile
  - Chest X-ray may show bilateral lung infiltrates
  - Patients may require supportive management with oxygen and ventilatory support

Options for patients refusing blood transfusion

- Some patients may refuse a blood transfusion for religious reasons, e.g. Jehovah's Witnesses
- Options include
  - Discuss if there are any blood components they would accept, even if they would not be willing to use packed red cells
  - Intraoperative cell salvage (collecting blood intraoperatively, mixing it with anticoagulant and re-transfusing the red blood cells intra- or post-operatively)
  - Preoperative autologous donation (patient donating units of their own blood pre-operatively in case the blood is needed intraoperatively)
- If none of the above are accepted, ensure that steps have been taken to maximise haemoglobin levels and minimise bleeding, such as
  - Replacement of iron, B12 and folate as required
  - Stopping NSAIDs, anticoagulant and antiplatelet therapies
  - Giving clotting agents such as tranexamic acid
  - Erythropoietin/darbepoetin – given as intravenous or subcutaneous injections to promote erythrocyte production

Mr Read receives another three units of packed red cells. His post-transfusion haemoglobin is 102 g/L. He is discharged after 1 week in hospital and given iron tablets to continue taking at home.

TIMEPOINT ⏱ 4

Four months later, Mr Read is brought to the emergency department. He called an ambulance as his ascites has been getting worse again, and today he has started to feel very unwell. He has been stable since he was last discharged from

Table 26.9 Venous blood results

White cell count	26.1×10^9/L	Urea	9.3 mmol/L
Haemoglobin	106 g/L	Creatinine	257 µmol/L
Platelets	354×10^9/L	Albumin	27 g/L
CRP	153 mg/L	Bilirubin	79 µmol/L
Sodium	131 mmol/L	Alkaline phosphatase	158 U/L
Potassium	5.8 mmol/L	Alanine aminotransferase	321 U/L

hospital. His course of antiviral treatment has finished, and his diuretic treatment was stopped when he was last discharged.

Over the last 72 hours his ascites has come back and his abdomen is becoming increasingly painful. He has been feeling hot and cold and cannot remember the last time he passed urine. He has not had any nausea or vomiting and his bowels have been opening normally.

His observations are:

Respiratory rate: 22/min
Oxygen saturations: 91% on room air
Temperature: 39.3°C
Blood pressure: 114/79 mmHg
Heart rate: 95 bpm

On examination he appears jaundiced, with significant abdominal distension. He also has pitting oedema to the knees bilaterally.

A urine dip does not show any evidence of infection, proteinuria or haematuria. Given his history, the emergency department doctor suspects spontaneous bacterial peritonitis so runs some initial blood tests (Table 26.9), as well as sending some ascitic fluid for analysis.

Based on the acutely deranged renal function, an ultrasound KUB is arranged which is completely normal.

What is the likeliest diagnosis? What are the criteria for this condition?

This picture could be explained by hepatorenal syndrome (HRS). HRS is the development of renal failure in a patient with decompensated liver disease, with no other identifiable cause of renal failure.

The criteria for diagnosis are:

- Serum creatinine >133 µmol/L
- Presence of cirrhosis and ascites
- No current/recent treatment with nephrotoxic drugs
- Absence of hypovolaemia
- Absence of shock
- Proteinuria <0.5 g/day, no microhaematuria and normal renal ultrasound

Types of HRS

Type 1 = Rapidly progressing acute renal failure. Usually triggered by a major event, e.g. variceal bleed or SBP. Associated with very low eGFR and poor prognosis. Creatinine doubles from baseline to >221 µmol/L.

Type 2 = Slowly progressing renal failure occurring in patient with refractory ascites and sodium retention. Can progress to type 1.

What is the management of hepatorenal syndrome?

- Close monitoring. Generally, patients should be managed on an HDU or ITU if possible
- Electrolyte abnormalities should be treated
- Patients should be screened for sepsis including urine, ascitic fluid and blood cultures and treated accordingly
- All diuretic and nephrotoxic medications should be stopped
- Terlipressin with albumin should be given as there is evidence that it improves renal function

- Liver transplantation is the definitive treatment. Prognosis of HRS is very poor (median survival time is 3 months). Many patients, especially those with type 1 HRS, do not survive the transplant waiting list

The ascitic fluid results confirm spontaneous bacterial peritonitis. Mr Read is moved to the high-dependency unit for closer monitoring, and he is started on ceftriaxone for the spontaneous bacterial peritonitis. He is also given treatment for his hyperkalaemia and hyponatraemia, and started on terlipressin with albumin. The consultant phones the hospital transplant coordinator and asks them to add Mr Read to the national waiting list for liver transplantation. Unfortunately, he continues to deteriorate despite treatment and passes away 3 days later from multi-organ failure.

Case 27

Mr Newman is a 53-year-old financial advisor who attends his GP as he has been having upper abdominal pain. His symptoms have been going on for a few months with intermittent pain, reflux, bloating and nausea. He finds that antacids used to work for him but are no longer making any difference. His past medical history includes mild depression, and he had a laparoscopic cholecystectomy for gallstone disease 10 years ago. He does not take any regular medications and is sensitive to tramadol. He smokes around 15 cigarettes a day and usually has 2 large glasses of red wine with dinner each night. He lives with his wife and their two cats. His BMI is 34, and he rarely gets to the gym as he works such long hours.

His observations are:

Respiratory rate: 18/min
Oxygen saturations: 99% on room air
Temperature: 36.1°C
Blood pressure: 127/73 mmHg
Heart rate: 83 bpm

Abdominal examination is unremarkable.

Which 'alarm' symptoms should the GP ask about?

'Alarm' or 'red flag' symptoms suggest that there may be a serious underlying cause of the dyspepsia and indicate that further investigation is likely to be required, usually with oesophagogastroduodenoscopy (OGD).

Symptoms which warrant urgent (2-week wait) referral include:

- Dysphagia
- Aged ≥55 plus weight loss, plus any of

- Upper abdominal pain
- Reflux
- Dyspepsia

Symptoms which warrant non-urgent referral include:

- Treatment-resistant dyspepsia
- Upper abdominal pain with low haemoglobin
- Melena
- Haematemesis
- Recurrent vomiting
- Iron-deficiency anaemia
- Epigastric mass
- Raised platelets with nausea/vomiting/weight loss/reflux/dyspepsia/upper abdominal pain
- Nausea or vomiting with weight loss/reflux/dyspepsia/upper abdominal pain

The GP asks Mr Newman whether he has any 'alarm' symptoms. Mr Newman denies all of these. The GP suggests that Mr Newman try a medication called omeprazole. Mr Newman asks how long he would need to take the medication for. The GP responds that it depends on how well it controls his symptoms, but if he responds well, he might need to take a lifelong maintenance dose.

Mr Newman says that he is not prepared to become reliant on medications and would like a different option. The GP suggests that he try making some lifestyle changes.

What lifestyle changes might the GP recommend?

- Eating smaller, more regular meals
- Weight loss if overweight
- Eating earlier in the day (i.e. not eating for at least 3 hours before bed)

DOI: 10.1201/9781351257725-27

- Tilting the bed so that the head is raised slightly
- Avoiding spicy, fatty and rich foods, or any other foods the patient thinks may be triggering their symptoms
- Cutting down on alcohol and caffeine consumption
- Stopping smoking

The GP also checks that Mr Newman doesn't have any repeat medications which might be problematic.

Which medications should patients with dyspepsia consider stopping?

Any medication which may cause dyspepsia or increases the risk of bleeding may be worthwhile stopping if the patient is at risk of or has peptic ulcer disease. In all cases, the risk–benefit profile must be carefully considered.

- Alpha-blockers
- Anticholinergics
- Anticoagulants
- Aspirin
- Benzodiazepines
- Beta-blockers
- Bisphosphonates
- Calcium channel blockers
- Metformin
- Nitrates
- NSAIDs
- SSRIs
- Steroids
- Theophyllines
- Tricyclic antidepressants

Mr Newman confirms that he does not have any repeat medications. He thanks the GP for the advice and says that he will try his best to follow it.

TIMEPOINT ⏱ 2

Three months later, Mr Newman returns to see his GP as his symptoms are worsening, despite trying all of the lifestyle measures suggested by the GP. The GP suggests testing for *Helicobacter pylori* as it is often associated with dyspepsia.

His observations are:

Respiratory rate: 16/min
Saturations: 98% on room air
Temperature: 37.2°C
Blood pressure: 133/79 mmHg
Heart rate: 74 bpm

Abdominal examination is unremarkable.

How can *H. pylori* be tested for?

- For all tests, the patient should not have used any acid suppression for 2 weeks prior or any antibiotics for 4 weeks prior as these may affect the test results
- All tests are highly sensitive and specific
- ^{13}C urea breath test
  - The patient drinks a drink containing urea with a labelled carbon isotope
  - If *H. pylori* is present the urea will be hydrolysed to ammonia and CO_2, meaning that the patient will breathe out labelled CO_2 after around 20 minutes which can be detected in breath samples
  - This can be used both to make a diagnosis and confirm eradication post-treatment
- Stool antigen test
  - The patient provides a stool sample which is tested for *H. pylori* antigen
  - This should not be used to confirm eradication
- Serology
  - For *H. pylori* IgG
  - Cannot reliably distinguish between current and previous infection
  - This is used less commonly than the non-invasive tests

Mr Newman agrees to have a ^{13}C urea breath test later in the week. The GP asks if anything else has changed since Mr Newman last attended. Mr Newman says that he has been taking lots of ibuprofen because of his arthritic knee pain, but nothing much else is different. The GP warns Mr

Newman that he should avoid NSAIDs if possible as they may make his symptoms worse.

What is the management of non-specific dyspepsia?

- Dyspepsia may be treated empirically with a 4-week course of a full-dose proton-pump inhibitor (PPI), for example
  - Esomeprazole 20 mg OD
  - Lansoprazole 30 mg OD
  - Omeprazole 20 mg OD
  - Pantoprazole 40 mg OD
- If reflux is predominant and GORD is suspected, treat with a PPI for 4–8 weeks
- If the response to the PPI is poor, an H_2 receptor antagonist may be given instead, such as ranitidine 150 mg BD
- For severe oesophagitis, it may also be necessary to give a double dose of PPI, or switch to a different one
- Consider whether it would be appropriate to test for *H. pylori*, and whether the patient has any red flags requiring a referral for urgent endoscopy
- Give *H. pylori* eradication treatment if confirmed by testing
- Patients who require long-term treatment should be reviewed annually
  - Advise them to consider reducing or stopping treatment, or returning to PRN treatment with over-the-counter antacids or alginates, if possible

Mr Newman has the ^{13}C urea breath test and is found to be *H. pylori*-positive. The GP phones him and asks him to come in and collect a prescription for eradication therapy.

What is used in eradication therapy for *H. pylori*?

H. pylori is eradicated with a 7-day course of triple therapy with a proton-pump inhibitor and a combination of two antibiotics, according to Table 27.1. If second-line treatment is not successful, the patient should be referred to gastroenterology.

TIMEPOINT ⏱ 3

Three years later, Mr Newman attends his GP again. He is now aged 56. When he last saw the GP, he had a good response to triple therapy with omeprazole, amoxicillin and clarithromycin. He has not used any treatment since, but unfortunately his symptoms have now started to come back again. He gets regular episodes of epigastric pain and nausea, but the predominant symptom is now reflux. He feels that the acid reflux is now much more severe than it was when his symptoms first started 3 years ago. He has no dysphagia or weight loss. He has spoken to a friend with similar symptoms and is worried that he may have a hiatus hernia as well.

His observations are:

Respiratory rate: 16/min
Oxygen saturations: 97% on room air

Table 27.1 *Helicobacter pylori* eradication therapies

	1: PPI	Triple therapy			
		First-line antibiotics		Second-line antibiotics	
		2: Antibiotic #1	3: Antibiotic #2	2: Antibiotic #1	3: Antibiotic #2
Penicillin safe	Esomeprazole 20 mg OD Lansoprazole 30 mg OD	Amoxicillin	Clarithromycin **OR** Metronidazole	Amoxicillin	Whichever antibiotic not used first line
Penicillin allergic	Omeprazole 20–40 mg OD Pantoprazole 40 mg OD	Clarithromycin	Metronidazole	Metronidazole	Levofloxacin

Temperature: 36.8°C
Blood pressure: 135/88 mmHg
Heart rate: 83 bpm

Abdominal examination is unremarkable.

What are the two types of hiatus hernia?

- Sliding
  - 85–95% of cases
  - The gastro-oesophageal junction slides above the diaphragm, into the thorax
  - These hernias may make GORD symptoms significantly worse
- Rolling (para-oesophageal)
  - 5–15% of cases
  - The gastro-oesophageal junction remains below the diaphragm, but part of the stomach rolls or folds through the diaphragm and sits above it, next to the oesophagus
  - Patients with these hernias are at risk of obstruction, ischaemia and volvulus (Figure 27.1)

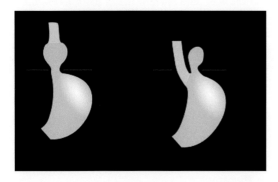

Figure 27.1 Left: sliding hernia. Right: rolling hernia.

The GP suggests that it might be worthwhile referring Mr Newman for an OGD. Mr Newman says that he feels very nervous about the idea of having a camera test and would like to know more about what it would involve.

What are the important risks of an OGD to warn a patient about when gaining their consent?

- Sore throat
- Damage to teeth
- Perforation +/− infection of the GI tract
- Bleeding (from biopsy site or damage to local structures)
- Reaction to sedatives such as allergy, hypotension or hypoventilation
- Aspiration pneumonia

Mr Newman has never had sedation before and asks the GP what it involves. He had been told by a friend that sedation is the same as having a general anaesthetic and wants to know if this is true.

What are the key messages about which to make the patient aware when explaining about pre-procedure sedation?

- Sedation is *not* the same as a general anaesthetic
- It may be suitable for a number of procedures including endoscopies, minor surgeries and biopsies
- It can be given orally or intravenously
- It makes you feel relaxed and less worried about the procedure that you will be having
- It may make you feel sleepy or drowsy. You will still be awake but you are unlikely to remember what happens in detail
- You should not require support for your breathing (unlike with a general anaesthetic) but will be monitored throughout
- Heavier sedation may require a couple of hours to wear off after the procedure, in which case you will be transferred to a recovery bay until you feel more awake
- Risks of sedation include slow breathing, low blood pressure, nausea, vomiting, having an allergic reaction, feeling unsteady or that it might have a temporary effect on your judgement, memory or decision-making
- Ensure the patient is aware that they cannot drive home safely. Ideally, they should not travel on public transport unaccompanied either. They will need someone to care for them and any dependents for 24 hours

- Nil by mouth rules: usually no food for 6 hours prior and no clear fluids for 2 hours prior
- For an OGD, the alternatives to sedation would include just using a local anaesthetic spray to numb the throat whilst remaining completely awake, or using a general anaesthetic. Another option would be to use the throat spray and the sedation together

Mr Newman is happy with the GP's explanations and agrees to the referral. The GP refers Mr Newman for a routine OGD. The OGD is normal, so the GP restarts Mr Newman on acid-suppression treatment (lansoprazole 30 mg OD) and asks him to come back if his symptoms worsen. He explains that he may need to take maintenance treatment long term to keep his symptoms under control. Mr Newman is happy with this.

TIMEPOINT ⏱ 4

One year later, Mr Newman returns to his GP, accompanied by his wife. He is now aged 57, and his symptoms are worse than ever. Despite good compliance with his lansoprazole treatment, he still has abdominal pain, reflux and dyspepsia on most days. Mr Newman thought there was no point going back to the doctor as he had a normal OGD last year, but his wife insisted as she was starting to worry about him. She tells the GP that she thinks it is strange that even though he is eating all the same meals as she is, he has lost a significant amount of weight this year. Mr Newman denies any dysphagia. The GP weighs him and notes that his weight is now 96 kg (BMI 31.3), compared to 104 kg when he was last weighed around 4 years ago.

His observations are:

Respiratory rate: 20/min
Oxygen saturations: 98% on room air
Temperature: 37.2°C
Blood pressure: 132/86 mmHg
Heart rate: 79 bpm

Abdominal examination is unremarkable, except for mild tenderness to palpation in the epigastric region.

The GP explains that given his symptoms in combination with his age and a history of weight loss, Mr Newman would qualify for a 2-week wait referral for another OGD to rule out the possibility of his symptoms being caused by an oesophageal cancer.

Mr Newman undergoes another OGD, during which biopsies are sent. The report says that there is 'evidence of columnar epithelium above the gastro-oesophageal junction'.

What is this condition known as, and what is the pathophysiology?

- This is known as Barrett's oesophagus
- It occurs when chronic acid reflux causes inflammation and erosion of the mucosa near the gastro-oesophageal junction, leading to the normal squamous epithelial lining undergoing metaplastic change to columnar epithelium
- This can be seen on OGD as the columnar epithelium has a red velvety appearance, compared to the pale and glossy normal squamous epithelium
- Biopsies should be taken to prove the diagnosis
- The risk of developing Barrett's oesophagus increases with duration of GORD
- Other risk factors include male gender, alcohol use, smoking, obesity and the presence of a hiatus hernia
- There is evidence to suggest that *H. pylori* infection and NSAID use may actually be protective
- Barrett's oesophagus is important as patients have a 40 times increased risk of developing oesophageal adenocarcinoma

Two weeks later, the GP receives a letter explaining that histology has confirmed that Mr Newman has Barrett's oesophagus. The GP calls Mr Newman in for an appointment to explain the diagnosis. The GP explains that he will now be added to the local surveillance programme.

How should surveillance be carried out for Barrett's oesophagus?

- This is a controversial area
- There is no specific surveillance regimen for patients with confirmed Barrett's oesophagus

- According to the British Society for Gastroenterology, it should depend on several factors, including
  - The size of the Barrett's segment
  - Estimated likelihood of cancer progression
  - Patient fitness for repeat endoscopy
  - Patient preference
- Usually, patients should have repeat endoscopy every 2–5 years, depending on the factors above
- Patients with symptoms of GORD alone should not be routinely screened
- Patients who have symptoms of GORD as well as certain risk factors (such as a family history in a first-degree relative, male gender, age above 50 years) may be considered for screening

If dysplasia is found on endoscopy, how is it managed?

- All cases of dysplasia should be discussed at an appropriate MDT
- Low-grade dysplasia is usually managed by endoscopy ablation with radiofrequency ablation
- High-grade dysplasia tends to use endoscopic resection of the visible abnormality, followed by endoscopic ablation
- More invasive cancers may require oesophagectomy
- Appropriate endoscopic follow-up should be arranged

Case 28

TIMEPOINT ⏱ 1

Ms Harris is a 19 year old who returned home from her gap year 6 days ago. She spent the year travelling around East and Southeast Asia.

She is brought to the GP by her mother who is concerned that she has been feverish over the last 48 hours. She tells the GP that she has a headache and feels that all her muscles ache, and she 'really doesn't feel good'. She hasn't noticed any other specific symptoms. She asks the GP to turn the lights off in the consulting room because they are very bright and making her eyes sore.

She had an appendicectomy aged 12 but has no other past medical or surgical history. She uses the combined pill for contraception and is still taking her antimalarial drug mefloquine, but otherwise she takes no regular medications. She has no drug allergies that she is aware of. She smokes 5–10 cigarettes a day and occasionally uses cannabis recreationally, but doesn't drink any alcohol.

On examination, her observations are:

Respiratory rate: 26/min
Oxygen saturations: 97% on room air
Temperature: 38.7°C
Blood pressure: 104/62 mmHg
Heart rate: 107 bpm

From the end of the bed she looks sweaty and appears unwell. Her extremities are cool, but she has a normal capillary refill time. Her cardiovascular, respiratory and abdominal examinations are otherwise normal. She has a reduced range of movement in her neck but there is no focal neurology. The GP cannot see any rashes.

What are the red flag clinical signs of meningitis?

- Petechial or purpuric rash, typically non-blanching
- Altered mental state
- Neck stiffness
- Photophobia
- Kernig's sign
- Brudzinski's sign
- Focal neurological defects
- Seizures

What tests might be performed in secondary care and why?

- Blood tests
  - Full blood count – to check for raised white cell count
  - CRP – if raised may be suggestive of infection
  - U&E and LFTs – as a baseline before antibiotic treatment
  - Blood cultures – to check for bacteraemia and to allow tailoring of antibiotics
  - PCR for *Neisseria meningitidis* – rapid test with high sensitivity and specificity for most common pathogen. Blood cultures are still gold standard, but PCR may be useful
- Cultures – to rule out alternative sources of infection
  - Urine
  - Nasal
  - Stool
- Imaging
  - Chest X-ray – to rule out a respiratory cause of the patient's deterioration

- Lumbar puncture
  - The patient has headache, fever, photophobia and neck stiffness
  - A lumbar puncture should be done unless contraindicated, for example if the patient has reduced GCS, severe headache or is fitting
  - Send samples for Gram stain, Ziehl–Neelsen staining, cytology, virology, glucose, protein, culture, antigen screen, PCR and India ink for cryptococci
  - Lumbar puncture may need repeating as it can be normal in early disease

What are the key causative organisms of meningitis?

- Bacterial
  - Neonates (under 3 months): Group B streptococci, *Escherichia coli*, *Listeria monocytogenes*
  - Children and adults: *Neisseria meningitidis*, *Haemophilus influenzae* type B, *Streptococcus pneumoniae*
  - Immunocompromised: *Listeria monocytogenes*
- Viral, for example herpesviruses, HIV, measles, mumps
- Fungal, for example Cryptococcus

The GP is concerned about the possibility of a bacterial meningitis.

He gives Ms Harris a stat dose of 1.2 g benzylpenicillin IM and calls 999 for an ambulance to transfer her to hospital urgently.

TIMEPOINT ⏱ 2

One hour later, Ms Harris arrives in resus and is given paracetamol and a stat bag of intravenous fluids.

Her observations one hour after this treatment are:

Respiratory rate: 24/min
Oxygen saturations: 96% on room air
Temperature: 37.8°C
Blood pressure: 119/73 mmHg
Heart rate: 101 bpm

Her observations are improving, and she appears to be clinically stable.

As she has already received a dose of benzylpenicillin, the emergency department doctor takes a more detailed history.

What are the key questions which should be asked in a travel history?

- History of presenting complaint, including details of time and location of onset and duration
- Details of travel history including locations visited, travel dates and methods of travel
- Types of location visited, e.g. urban, forest, mountains, rural
- Purpose of travel and activities undertaken, e.g. healthcare or emergency aid workers more likely to come into contact with disease or poor living conditions
- If the patient has had contact with animals and insects (whether or not they recall being bitten or scratched)
- If the patient has had unprotected sexual intercourse or injected intravenous drugs
- Whether the patient received all the required vaccinations and prophylaxis prior to travelling
- What foods the patient ate, how these were prepared and whether the patient may have come into contact with unsafe drinking water
- Whether the patient had contact with the healthcare system abroad and details of this, for example if they may have come into contact with non-sterile equipment, if they received medications or blood products which might be infected

Ms Harris confirms that her symptoms only started 48 hours ago, approximately 4 days after her return flight from Shanghai airport. She spent 8 months travelling around Thailand, Vietnam, Indonesia and China. This included urban, forested and mountain regions. During the final 3 months of her trip, she worked in an animal sanctuary in the Chinese forests. She doesn't recall sustaining any bites or scratches from any animal she worked with or any insects. She slept under an insect net and used insect repellent daily. She tried to wear long clothes most of the time, although sometimes she felt it was too hot and wore outfits which did not cover her skin as fully. She denies having unprotected intercourse during the trip or using any intravenous drugs. She insists that she was very careful to use water-purification tablets with all of her drinking water, but she was sometimes tempted by street food because she was keen to try local delicacies.

She reports that she received all the recommended vaccinations prior to her trip, including all the additional ones recommended as she stated that she was planning to work outdoors with animals (hepatitis A, hepatitis B, Japanese encephalitis, tetanus booster, rabies, tick-borne encephalitis and typhoid). She took her malaria prophylaxis as prescribed and doesn't recall missing any doses. She did not attend any local healthcare services during her time abroad as she took a full year's supply of her contraceptive pill and malaria prophylaxis, and has otherwise been well.

What are the key differential diagnoses which should be considered in an unwell returning traveller?

See Table 28.1.

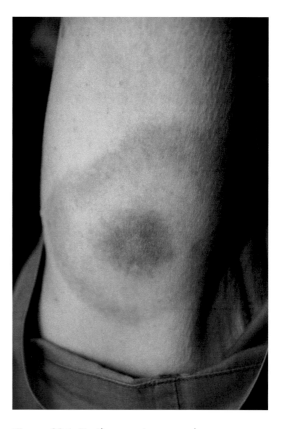

Figure 28.1 Erythema migrans rash.

On closer examination, the emergency department doctor discovers a blanching rash which was hidden by Ms Harris' hair. The rash is not itchy or painful.

The emergency department doctor concludes that the likeliest diagnosis is Lyme disease, given her possible exposure to tick bites whilst working near animals in the Chinese forests, and the typical erythema migrans rash (Figure 28.1) that she has developed.

He sends further blood tests to check for Lyme disease serum antibodies and also requests a malaria screen (thick and thin Giemsa stained blood films).

Table 28.1 Key differential diagnoses for an unwell returning traveller

	Aetiology/ locations	Incubation period	Fever	Headache	Myalgia	Cough	Nausea and vomiting	Jaundice	Rash	Diarrhoea	Hepatomegaly	Splenomegaly	Other
Chikungunya fever	Virus transmitted via mosquitoes in Africa, Southeast Asia, America	4–8 days	Y						Y				#1
Cholera	*Vibrio cholerae* in fecally contaminated water, in Africa, Asia, Middle East and South America	2–5 days								Y			
Dengue fever	Virus transmitted by Aedes mosquitoes in Southeast Asia, Southern Europe, North America	Up to 2 weeks	Y	Y	Y		Y		Y				
Hepatitis A	Virus transmitted via fecal-oral route in Indian subcontinent, Africa, Far East, South and Central America, Middle East	2–6 weeks	Y				Y	Y	Y		Y	Y	
Lyme disease	*Borrelia* spp. via Ixodes ticks in Europe, USA and Asia	3–30 days	Y						Y				#2
Malaria	*Plasmodium* spp. carried by Anopheles mosquitoes in tropics and subtropics	7–40 days	Y	Y	Y	Y	Y	Y	Y	Y	Y	Y	
Rabies	Virus transmitted via saliva in infected animal bites, worldwide	3–12 weeks (rarely years)	Y	Y									#3
Typhoid	*Salmonella typhi* in Africa and Asia, from contaminated water	10–20 days	Y	Y		Y			Y	Y			#4

(Continued)

Table 28.1 (Continued) Key differential diagnoses for an unwell returning traveller

Aetiology/ locations	Incubation period	Fever	Headache	Myalgia	Cough	Nausea and vomiting	Jaundice	Rash	Diarrhoea	Hepatomegaly	Splenomegaly	Other
Typhus	Rickettsia spp., transmitted by contamination of wounds with infected louse feces	10–14 days	Y	Y	Y	Y	Y		Y	Y			#5
Viral haemorrhagic fevers	Including Ebola virus, Lassa fever, Zika virus, via animal/ mosquito vectors in Africa, Asia and Europe	2–21 days	Y	Y	Y	Y	Y						#6
West Nile virus	Virus transmitted via mosquitoes in Africa, Europe, Middle East, Asia, North America	2–14 days	Y	Y	Y						Y	Y	#7
Yellow fever	Virus transmitted via mosquitoes in South America and Sub-Saharan Africa	3–6 days	Y	Y	Y		Y	Y					#8

#1 = severe polyarthritis
#2 = flu-like symptoms, facial nerve palsies, meningitis, encephalitis, arthritis
#3 = pain and paraesthesiae at wound site, weakness in affected limb, altered mental state (agitation, delirium), hydrophobia, difficulty swallowing, focal neurological signs, paralysis
#4 = epistaxis, Faget's sign (relative bradycardia)
#5 = gangrene/necrosis of extremities
#6 = signs of vascular damage, e.g. conjunctival injection, petechial haemorrhage, mucous membrane haemorrhage
#7 = flu-like symptoms
#8 = DIC, AKI

Serological testing in Lyme disease

- In a patient who has travelled from a Lyme-endemic region, a clinical diagnosis of Lyme disease can be made based on the typical erythema migrans rash, with no need for serological testing
- If there is clinical suspicion of Lyme disease without erythema migrans, consider serology testing and consider starting antibiotics without waiting for results
- Testing at the time of presentation gives a high chance of false negative results as the antibodies take time to develop and the test has a low sensitivity
- If there is doubt, the test can be repeated at 3–4 weeks post-initial presentation
- The test works best for *Borrelia burgforderi* and may not detect other strains
- Discuss with your infectious disease specialist or microbiologist if you are considering testing

Ms Harris is started on a 3-week course of intravenous ceftriaxone and remains in hospital to complete the course.

What practical steps should be taken if a patient attends with a possible tropical infection?

- Appropriate infection control depending on method of transmission, for example
  - Hand hygiene
  - Personal protective equipment such as masks, eye protection
  - Contact precautions: wearing of aprons and gloves
  - Airborne/droplet precautions: isolation in negative pressure side room, masks, respirators
- Discussion with infection control team, or local tropical disease service

Is Lyme disease a notifiable disease? Which diseases are notifiable in UK?

Lyme disease is not notifiable in the UK.

However, acute meningitis, meningococcal septicaemia or a confirmed case of *Neisseria meningitidis* would all be notifiable to Public Health England.

Many of the other differential diagnoses which should be considered in a returning traveller *are* notifiable.

List of notifiable diseases

- Acute encephalitis
- Acute infectious hepatitis
- Acute meningitis
- Acute poliomyelitis
- Anthrax
- Botulism
- Brucellosis
- Cholera
- Diphtheria
- Enteric fever (typhoid or paratyphoid fever)
- Food poisoning
- Haemolytic uraemic syndrome (HUS)
- Infectious bloody diarrhoea
- Invasive group A streptococcal disease
- Legionnaires' disease
- Leprosy
- Malaria
- Measles
- Meningococcal septicaemia
- Mumps
- Plague
- Rabies
- Rubella
- Severe acute respiratory syndrome (SARS)
- Scarlet fever
- Smallpox
- Tetanus
- Tuberculosis
- Typhus
- Viral haemorrhagic fever (VHF)
- Whooping cough
- Yellow fever

List of notifiable organisms

- *Bacillus anthracis*
- *Bacillus cereus* (only if associated with food poisoning)
- *Bordetella pertussis*
- *Borrelia* spp.
- *Brucella* spp.
- *Burkholderia mallei*
- *Burkholderia pseudomallei*
- *Campylobacter* spp.
- Chikungunya virus
- *Chlamydophila psittaci*
- *Clostridium botulinum*
- *Clostridium perfringens* (only if associated with food poisoning)
- *Clostridium tetani*
- *Corynebacterium diphtheriae*
- *Corynebacterium ulcerans*
- *Coxiella burnetii*
- Crimean–Congo haemorrhagic fever virus
- *Cryptosporidium* spp.
- Dengue virus
- Ebola virus
- *Entamoeba histolytica*
- *Francisella tularensis*
- *Giardia lamblia*
- Guanarito virus
- *Haemophilus influenzae* (invasive)
- Hanta virus
- Hepatitis A, B, C, delta and E viruses
- Influenza virus
- Junin virus
- Kyasanur Forest disease virus
- Lassa virus
- *Legionella* spp.
- *Leptospira interrogans*
- *Listeria monocytogenes*
- Machupo virus
- Marburg virus
- Measles virus
- Mumps virus
- Mycobacterium tuberculosis complex
- *Neisseria meningitidis*
- Omsk haemorrhagic fever virus
- *Plasmodium falciparum, vivax, ovale, malariae, knowlesi*
- Polio virus (wild or vaccine types)
- Rabies virus (classical rabies and rabies-related lyssaviruses)
- *Rickettsia* spp.
- Rift Valley fever virus
- Rubella virus
- Sabia virus
- *Salmonella* spp.
- SARS coronavirus
- *Shigella* spp.
- *Streptococcus pneumoniae* (invasive)
- *Streptococcus pyogenes* (invasive)
- Varicella zoster virus
- Variola virus
- Verocytotoxigenic *Escherichia coli* (including *E. coli* O157)
- *Vibrio cholerae*
- West Nile virus
- Yellow fever virus
- *Yersinia pestis*

TIMEPOINT ⏱ 3

Ten days later, Ms Harris is being reviewed on the morning medical ward round when the consultant notices that she is unable to smile properly. She has noticed that loud noises have been particularly painful over the last 24 hours. She denies any changes to her sense of taste.

On examination, her observations are:

Respiratory rate: 18/min
Oxygen saturations: 98% on room air
Temperature: 36.2°C
Blood pressure: 121/84 mmHg
Heart rate: 73 bpm

From the end of the bed, she appears well but has a clear droop on the left side of her mouth.

On examination, she is unable to raise her left eyebrow, close her left eye tightly or blow out her left cheek. The right side of her face appears to be completely unaffected.

No abnormality is detected on otoscopy, and the inside of the mouth, including the palate and the tongue, all appear normal. There are no rashes on her face.

Her cranial nerve examination is otherwise normal.

Her upper and lower limb neurological examinations are also normal.

The consultant suspects that she has developed a facial nerve (cranial nerve VII) palsy.

- **Upper motor neurone lesions =** forehead sparing
- **Lower motor neurone lesions =** forehead is affected; therefore patient is unable to raise eyebrows

---

How can a facial nerve palsy secondary to Lyme disease be distinguished from a Bell's palsy?

- Bell's palsy refers to an idiopathic facial nerve palsy; therefore by definition it is a diagnosis of exclusion
- Facial nerve palsy secondary to Lyme disease is commonly misdiagnosed as Bell's palsy
- This is significant as the management may differ between the two
- If the palsy recurs or is bilateral, it is likely to be related to Lyme disease

What are the other differential diagnoses for a facial nerve palsy?

- Idiopathic (Bell's palsy)
  - Significantly more common in diabetic and pregnant patients
- Iatrogenic, e.g. secondary to local anaesthetic infiltration
- Infective causes
  - Viruses, e.g. Cytomegalovirus, Epstein–Barr virus, HIV, Herpes simplex virus 1
  - Varicella Zoster virus (HSV3), also known as Ramsay Hunt syndrome
- Stroke
- Trauma, e.g. skull base fracture
- Malignancy, e.g. parotid gland or posterior fossa tumours
- Multiple sclerosis
- Guillain–Barré syndrome

What is the management of a facial nerve palsy secondary to Lyme disease?

- Continue the course of antibiotics as prescribed
- Eye care
  - Artificial tears/eye drops/ointments
  - Eye patch
  - Occasionally Botox or surgery is needed to protect the eye
- Steroids are sometimes given
  - Controversial area
  - In Bell's palsy, steroids should be given if the patient presents within 72 hours of onset
  - However, in facial nerve palsy secondary to Lyme disease there is recent evidence to suggest that giving steroids leads to worse outcomes
- Consider whether referrals to neurology, ENT, ophthalmology or plastic surgery are needed

TIMEPOINT ⏱ 4

Four weeks after her discharge from the medical ward, Ms Harris presents to the emergency department with a 2-day history of profuse watery diarrhoea and abdominal cramping. She reports that she has opened her bowels five times in the last 24 hours. All of the stools have been very watery (type 6–7).

On examination, her observations are:

Respiratory rate: 20/min
Oxygen saturations: 95% on room air
Temperature: 37.2°C
Blood pressure: 126/91 mmHg
Heart rate: 84 bpm

Her cardiovascular and respiratory examinations are within normal limits. Her abdomen is soft, with mild tenderness to palpation in all quadrants but with no signs of peritonism. Bowel sounds are normal.

Bloods tests show:

Venous blood results

White cell count	14.2×10^9/L
CRP	38 mg/L
Haemoglobin	122 g/L
Urea	4.7 mmol/L
Creatinine	98 μmol/L
Lactate	0.9 mmol/L

What is the most likely diagnosis and what is the cause of this?

Certain antibiotics may cause pseudomembranous (entero)colitis. This is when antibiotics lead to the destruction of the normal gut flora, allowing *Clostridium difficile* to superinfect the colon, resulting in severe diarrhoea. It is usually secondary to long-term treatment with broad-spectrum antibiotics.

Commonly implicated classes of antibiotics include cephalosporins, fluoroquinolones, macrolides and beta lactam-beta lactamase inhibitor combined agents such as clavulanic acid-amoxicillin (co-amoxiclav) or piperacillin-tazobactam (tazocin).

How should it be managed?

- Send stool samples to test for *Clostridium difficile* toxin
- Correct fluid loss and electrolyte imbalances as required
- Stop the antibiotics if possible, or consider changing to an antibiotic less likely to cause pseudomembranous (entero)colitis
- Avoid using drugs which may slow peristalsis, for example codeine or loperamide
- Metronidazole, vancomycin or fidaxomin may be used as therapy
- Surgical intervention may rarely be required in cases of severe colitis
- Report confirmed cases to Public Health England

FURTHER READING

1. https://www.ncbi.nlm.nih.gov/pmc/articles/PMC3640964/
2. https://www.sciencedirect.com/science/article/pii/S1877959X1730167X
3. https://www.gov.uk/guidance/lyme-disease-sample-testing-advice
4. https://www.gov.uk/guidance/notifiable-diseases-and-causative-organisms-how-to-report
5. https://www.nice.org.uk/guidance/ng95/chapter/Recommendations#laboratory-investigations-to-support-diagnosis
6. www.ncbi.nlm.nih.gov/pubmed/27598389.

Case 29

Mr Woll, a 43-year-old shop assistant, went on holiday to Zimbabwe predominantly aiming to see animals on safari. He had experienced mild toothache for 2 days before the flight but reassured himself it was not severe enough to change carefully booked travel plans. However, 3 days after arriving, the pain has become nearly unbearable, and he seeks a local dentist. The work needed is major, requiring significant use of sharp equipment. During the procedure, the dentist unfortunately injures himself, then hastily finishes the procedure and tells Mr Woll that he will need to undergo some blood tests. Later, documentation provided via the dentist reveals that he had breached regulator guidelines and worked whilst knowingly HIV-positive.

The traveller Mr Woll is very perplexed by what needs to be done, and it takes several hours to navigate the local healthcare systems, and eventually he is sent to a location for blood tests. He fears acquisition of hepatitis and/or HIV but no post-exposure prophylaxis is available. Mr Woll has no significant past medical history and does not take any regular medications. He has mild hayfever but is not aware of any other allergies. He has never smoked and drinks occasionally when socialising. He usually lives with his partner, although she had not accompanied him on this holiday due to business commitments.

What is post-exposure prophylaxis?

Very well-conducted research and observational studies have shown a dramatic reduction in risk of acquisition of HIV when medication taken soon after exposure is administered, based on the theory that HIV can be prevented from ongoing infection by doing so. Post-exposure prophylaxis (PEP) is a combination treatment which should be initiated as soon as possible, ideally within 2 hours, and most probably within a limited time frame. It is effective; the rate of infection is reduced by approximately 80%, compared to when PEP is not used.

TIMEPOINT ⏱ 2

Three hours later, Mr Woll feels desperate and fears acquisition of communicable viral pathogens could have taken place. He asks everyone he can find how and where to seek expert advice. He finally is advised to attend a clinic where, with significant sensitivity, care and thought, the likely risk of conversion to HIV seropositivity is communicated. This is rather nuanced given the dental environment in which the incident took place and the imprecise knowledge to provide a quantifiable risk; however, given the HIV status of the dentist and the understandable concern generated, careful notes are taken and the presumed professional and governance issues related to the dentist would be looked into on a future occasion. There is extremely irregular availability of post-exposure prophylactic medication in that region of Zimbabwe, and on this occasion, it is not possible to get a supply to him in the days that follow.

Which countries have relatively high HIV prevalence?

The following countries are estimated to have a >10% HIV prevalence: Swaziland, Lesotho, Botswana, South Africa, Namibia, Zimbabwe, Zambia, Mozambique.

TIMEPOINT ⏱ 3

Twelve days later, back in the UK, Mr Woll develops a feverish, unpleasant illness; he notes that his glands are up and for several days has to take paracetamol, drink lots of fluids and keep off work. He knows in his own mind that this probably represents primary/seroconverting illness, and he attends a large NHS hospital in Central London, where those thoughts are confirmed. Given all the background, he then has intensive blood tests both immediately and in the days that follow, and when the (not unexpected) result of HIV positivity is confirmed, anti-retroviral medication is started and regular telephone and outpatient follow-up arranged.

What is HIV seroconversion illness/ acute HIV infection?

This description is of a very common illness that takes place from a few days up until several months after HIV exposure. It manifests in a variety of ways but shares some features of other severe viral clinical syndromes. Rash, myalgia, fatigue and a high fever are common, and the temperature reached is usually between 38 and 40°C. Other generalised features include lymphadenopathy, gastrointestinal symptoms and neurological aspects such as headache and possibly a form of aseptic meningitis. The condition resolves by itself, but in the presence of a high index of suspicion should prompt (1) testing to ascertain HIV status and (2) an awareness of a possible period of high levels of HIV viraemia.

What is the differential diagnosis of acute HIV infection?

A wide range of conditions, infective and non-infective, can present in a quite similar manner; they include CMV, EBV, viral hepatitis, relapsing fevers, Ebola, adult-onset Still's disease, SLE, etc.

Reducing HIV transmission

There have been major and, for the most part, successful education and interventional efforts to reduce the level of HIV transmission across the world.

There are four methods via which transmission may take place: two within the healthcare setting and two in the non-healthcare setting.

- Blood products
  - Pre-testing and screening of the products are very effective
- Exposure prone procedures
  - The 'recipient' in the relevant incident(s) will be advised to seek immediate healthcare in order to perform procedures to reduce risk and also to consider if post-exposure prophylactic medication is indicated
- Close personal contact
  - A combination of education and suitable methods alongside the possibility – where relevant – of pre-exposure prophylaxis are possible
- Vertical transmission – from mother to fetus/baby
  - Testing of pregnant women
  - Where needed antiretroviral treatment
  - Careful selection of mode of delivery (e.g. Caesarean section) and prophylactic measures
  - Bottle feeding for the baby

TIMEPOINT ⏱ 4

One year later, Mr Woll is reviewed in his local university hospital HIV clinic. He has complete confidence in their ability to monitor and work with him on adjusting his ongoing HIV-related medication. He has a CD4 count within the reference range, an undetectable viral load and liver function, renal function, haemoglobin and lipid profile at or very near to target levels. He plans to contribute to a charity fund to help with combined patient and professional educational events being put together via his clinical team and aims to continue follow-up in the current clinic.

HIV treatments and their side effects

It barely does justice to provide this very brief overview of categories that outline the current range of anti-HIV medical treatments. There is an immense published literature on this subject. Within 2–3 decades of fully being recognised, HIV therapy has seen the outcome of this condition change from a high fatality rate to an immeasurably different condition – where effective treatment can be obtained, meaning living with HIV as a chronic condition is commonplace. Dedicated in-depth research has unlocked molecular mechanisms to help understand the machinery of the virus, thus providing the keys to several kinds of antiretroviral drugs. The precise timing of initiating and reviewing and combination treatment is individualised and subject to local protocol, but the broad medication categories include:

- Nucleoside reverse transcriptase inhibitors (NRTI)
- Non-nucleoside reverse transcriptase inhibitors (NNRTI)
- Protease inhibitors
- Integrase inhibitors
- CCR5 receptor antagonists

Common side effects include lipid and glucose disorders, lipodystrophy, skin rashes, gastrointestinal conditions, liver dysfunction and blood disorders.

Why are lipid disorders related to HIV medication so important?

There is extensive evidence that anti-HIV medications are linked with dyslipidaemia and other metabolic alterations. Given that they are taken for long durations, and the potential presence of other cardiovascular risk factors, it means HIV medication monitoring and risk of cardiovascular events are key features of managing HIV-related treatment. Adipose redistribution is a key issue. Subcutaneous fat is often found in an altered pattern from the face and extremities to the trunk, neck, breasts and abdomen – which is frequently highly noticeable and may be distressing to patients.

FURTHER READING

1. http://arv.ashm.org.au/what-to-start-initial-combination-regimens-for-the-antiretroviral-naive-patient/

Case 30

Ms Jones, a 32-year-old marketing consultant, attends her GP with a 5-week history of feeling tired all the time, despite sleeping significantly more than she used to. She says that she feels exhausted all day long, even though she now gets around 10 hours sleep compared to her previously managing fine with 6.

She is worried about her work as she feels that she is letting her team down by not being as good at her job as she was before. She finds it difficult to concentrate during meetings and has missed several important deadlines over the last month. In her spare time, she used to enjoy baking with her daughter, but lately she has found that she is not interested in this and would rather go to sleep.

She denies any attempts at suicide or self-harm but admits she sometimes wonders whether her family would be better off without her.

On examination, her observations are normal. Her general examination is unremarkable although the doctor notes that her clothes appear to fit loosely. On further questioning she reveals that she has dropped two dress sizes due to weight loss over the last 3 months.

Ms Jones has a past medical history of psoriasis and irritable bowel syndrome. For her skin, she uses emollients regularly and adds in Dovobet (calipotriol/betamethasone) when she has flares. She is able to manage her IBS herself with a combination of laxatives and peppermint oil capsules as needed. She has no known drug allergies. She lives with her partner and 4-year-old daughter. She drinks around 20 units of alcohol a week and has never smoked.

What are diagnostic criteria for depression (according to NICE and DSM-IV/V: major depressive disorder)?

Core symptoms

- Loss of interest/pleasure in activities previously enjoyed (anhedonia)
- Persistent low mood

Secondary symptoms

- Change in sleep pattern – excessive sleepiness or insomnia
- Indecisiveness or inability to concentrate
- Change in weight and/or change in appetite
- Lack of energy or fatigue
- Excessive guilt or feelings of worthlessness
- Psychomotor agitation or retardation
- Suicidal ideation or attempts

Patients must display five or more of the above symptoms, including at least one of the core symptoms.

The symptoms must occur for most of the day, nearly every day, for at least 2 weeks, and be causing distress to the patient.

The symptoms must not be attributable to any other medical condition or medication.

Severity criteria

- Mild severity: five symptoms with minimal social/occupational impairment
- Moderate: five+ core symptoms with variable social/occupational impairment
- Severe: five+ core symptoms with significant social/occupational impairment

Table 30.1 Management options for treatment of depression

	Mild–moderate	Moderate–severe
First line	Watchful waiting OR low-intensity psychological interventions	SSRI AND psychological intervention
Second line	SSRIs	If SSRIs not tolerated, consider alternative, e.g. tricyclic antidepressant
Third line	If SSRIs not tolerated, consider alternative, e.g. tricyclic antidepressant	Electroconvulsive therapy

With all interventions, review the patient after 2 weeks to assess progress.

What would be the first- and second-line options for treatment?

Ms Jones would be classified as having moderate–severe depression (Table 30.1).

Low-intensity psychological interventions

- Guided self-help cognitive behavioural therapy
- Computerised cognitive behavioural therapy
- Relaxation therapy

Psychological interventions

- Cognitive behavioural therapy
- Interpersonal therapy

Selective serotonin reuptake inhibitors (SSRIs)

- e.g. fluoxetine, sertraline, citalopram
- Warn patient about risk of bleeding and other side effects, e.g. gastrointestinal upset
- Check for drug interactions, e.g. St John's Wort, aspirin, clopidogrel
- Make sure the patient is aware that it will take time for the treatment to work fully (up to 8 weeks)
- Make sure the patient is aware not to stop treatment suddenly (risk of SSRI discontinuation syndrome)

TIMEPOINT ⏱ 2

Ten days later, Ms Jones is brought into the local emergency department by her partner, who reports that he came home from work at 7.30 pm to find her sprawled on the bed, surrounded by tissues and an empty paracetamol packet.

She says that she took a few tablets early in the morning because she had a headache, but after that she was feeling so down that she kept taking tablets until she had finished an entire packet of 16 tablets over the next couple of hours. She denies taking them with any alcohol or any other medications.

Her observations are normal and there is nothing to find on examination.

She complains of feeling nauseous so is prescribed some anti-emetics.

What questions do you need to ask for any overdose or poisoning history?

- Regarding the drug taken
  - What time was the drug taken?
  - Which drugs were taken?
  - How many tablets were taken/what were the quantities?
  - Were the drugs taken with alcohol?
- Depression history: including all core and secondary symptoms
- Suicide risk assessment, as below

What are the components of a suicide risk assessment?

- What led up to the attempt? What was the tipping point or trigger?
- Have they made any previous attempts at suicide or self-harm?

- What was the method of attempted suicide? When and where did they to it? How were they discovered?
- Were alcohol or drugs involved?
- Was it a spontaneous attempt, or had they made plans in advance? Advance plans might include: stockpiling medications, writing a suicide note, making precautions to avoid being found by others, preparing a will or dealing with finances
- How do they feel now? Do they feel sad, angry or regretful? Would they attempt suicide again now if they had the opportunity?
- Do they have any protective factors? What do they have to live for?

What features would make this overdose high risk?

- Staggered overdose
- Overdose taken with alcohol
- Overdose taken with an additional drug

- High-dose overdose (over 150 mg paracetamol per kg weight)

How should Ms Jones be managed?

- Consider giving activated charcoal if the patient attends within 1 hour of ingestion of >150 mg/kg paracetamol
- If on or above the treatment line (Figure 30.1), give N-acetylcysteine (NAC) = 3× back-to-back infusions
  - Bag 1 = 150 mg/kg NAC (max 16.5 g) in 200 mL 5% glucose or 0.9% NaCl over 1 hour
  - Bag 2 = 50 mg/kg NAC (max 5.5 g) in 500 mL 5% glucose or 0.9% NaCl over 4 hours
  - Bag 3 = 100 mg/kg NAC (max 11 g) in 1000 mL 5% glucose or 0.9% NaCl over 16 hours
- Consider intensive care and psychiatric referrals

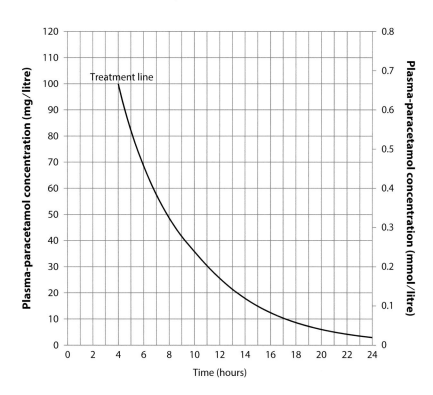

Figure 30.1 Treatment line graph for paracetamol overdose.

> **Key point**
>
> Use of the treatment line does not apply in staggered overdose – all staggered overdoses should be treated with NAC.

TIMEPOINT ⏱ 3

Ms Jones is treated with N-acetylcysteine as per protocol and moved to the acute medical unit overnight. Twelve hours later, Ms Jones' partner arrives to visit her. He shows the doctors a picture of four empty wine bottles which he had found hidden under the kitchen sink and then goes in to see her. Ms Jones is asleep when he arrives. He wakes her up to say hello, but she is very drowsy. She opens her eyes slightly, and he immediately notices that her eyes appear yellow. He goes to fetch a nurse who calls for the doctor.

Ms Jones' blood tests are repeated, including an arterial blood gas (Table 30.2).

What does the ABG show?

The ABG shows evidence of a raised anion gap metabolic acidosis. This could also be classified as a Type B2 lactic acidosis (Table 30.3).

What are the criteria for liver transplantation?

The most commonly used criteria are the King's College Criteria, which are as follows:

Patients should be referred for liver transplant immediately if they have:

- Arterial pH <7.3

OR all three of the following:

- INR>6.5 or PT>100
- Creatinine >300
- Grade III/IV hepatic encephalopathy

Table 30.2 Venous and arterial blood results

Venous blood tests	
White cell count	8.0×10^9/L
Haemoglobin	124 g/L
Platelets	297×10^9/L
Sodium	142 mmol/L
Potassium	4.3 mmol/L
Urea	6.4 mmol/L
Creatinine	420 µmol/L
INR	7.2
Bilirubin	92 µmol/L
Alanine aminotransferase	1734 u/L
Alkaline phosphatase	143 u/L
Albumin	37 g/L
Arterial blood gas	
pH	6.92
$PaCO_2$	3.9 kPa
PaO_2	10.5 kPa
HCO_3	5.8 mmol/L
Base excess	−23.9 mmol/L
Lactate	8.4 mmol/L
Sodium	142 mmol/L
Potassium	4.2 mmol/L
Chloride	101 mmol/L

Ms Jones qualifies for a liver transplant and is transferred to the local transplant centre. She has the transplant and is started on tacrolimus, azathioprine and prednisolone. She recovers well from the operation and is discharged from hospital 2 weeks later once her liver function tests have normalised.

TIMEPOINT ⏱ 4

Two months later, Ms Jones attends her liver specialist for a follow-up appointment. Prior to the appointment, she was asked to have blood tests, the results of which are given in Table 30.4.

Ms Jones denies any symptoms, and her observations and abdominal examination are normal.

Table 30.3 Types and causes of lactic acidosis

Type of lactic acidosis		Causes
A (Secondary to hypoperfusion and hypoxia, causing anaerobic glycolysis)		Shock (septic, cardiogenic, or any other type) Ischaemia Seizure Carbon monoxide poisoning
B (Not related to hypoperfusion and hypoxia)	1 (Associated with underlying disease)	Malignancy Infection Liver failure Renal failure Pancreatitis Diabetic ketoacidosis
	2 (Related to drugs or toxins)	Paracetamol Salicylates Methanol Metformin
	3 (Inborn errors of metabolism)	G6PD deficiency Pyruvate decarboxylase deficiency

What could be causing these blood test results?

- Acute cellular rejection occurs in up to 50% of patients within one year of liver transplantation
- It is usually asymptomatic and picked up due to deranged LFTs
- The diagnosis is confirmed by liver biopsy
- Treatment is using a short course of high-dose steroids, after which the patient's usual immunosuppression regime is increased
- Chronic rejection may occur if the patient has recurrent acute rejection, or acute rejection that is refractory to treatment

Ms Jones is admitted to the hepatology ward for a liver biopsy and further monitoring. Liver biopsy confirms acute cellular rejection and Ms Jones is started on high-dose steroids. Her usual immunosuppression regime is altered. After 1 week, her LFTs have normalised again, and the consultant is happy to discharge her.

What other complications are there of liver transplantation, other than acute cellular rejection?

- Hyperacute rejection
  - Rare unless donor ABO-incompatible
  - Due to pre-formed antibodies against donor major histocompatibility complex
  - Causes massive hepatic necrosis occurring within days
- Chronic rejection
  - Occurs after months to years

Table 30.4 Venous blood results

White cell count	6.3 × 10⁹/L	Urea	6.7 mmol/L
Haemoglobin	131 g/L	Creatinine	89 µmol/L
Platelets	346 × 10⁹/L	Albumin	34 g/L
MCV	87 fL	Bilirubin	36 µmol/L
Sodium	137 mmol/L	Alkaline phosphatase	178 U/L
Potassium	4.9 mmol/L	Alanine aminotransferase	102 U/L

- Usually presents with progressive cholestasis
- In later stages bile duct loss and fibrosis are seen
- Treatment is with escalation of immunosuppression or re-transplantation
- Graft failure
  - Transplant does not start working properly
- Bleeding
  - Liver transplantation is particularly high risk as patients may have clotting deficiencies secondary to the liver failure
- Post-operative wound infection, opportunistic infection secondary to use of immunosuppressive medications, and malignancy
- Transplanted patients are heavily immunosuppressed so at high risk
- Post-transplant lymphoproliferative disorder
- Thrombosis of the vena cava, portal vein or hepatic artery
- Biliary anastomotic leak
- Biliary strictures
  - Secondary to poor preservation of the liver during the transplantation procedure
- Disease recurrence
  - Hepatitis B, hepatitis C, alcoholic liver disease, PBC, PSC and autoimmune hepatitis have all been documented as having recurred in a transplanted liver

Case 31

Mr Roberts is a 64 year old who works as a registrar for births, marriages and deaths who has found the last 2 years the hardest of his otherwise unblemished 34-year career, partly connected to his closest colleague leaving to move to Canada. He has found he has been working unpaid extra hours – and work thus has felt immensely stressful. He has experienced several relatives passing away, was divorced 4 years ago and felt this work would help him sort out his financial affairs. He has become increasingly lonely and rarely visits the GP. Mr Roberts was usually fit and well with no past medical history, but he has taken a total of 11 sick days in the month leading up to his hospital admission.

On the day of admission, the neighbour comes out of her house, and is surprised because Mr Roberts usually turns on his favourite radio 'talk show' immediately after starting his car to drive to work; it seems his car has been running for a very long time inside the garage, but she hears no voices from the radio.

She calls the police in case something is wrong. They arrive, crank up the garage door, see tubing from the exhaust to the driver and immediately call an ambulance.

On arrival Mr Roberts has the following features:

Respiratory rate: 29/min
Oxygen saturations: 99% on room air
Temperature: 36.5°C
Blood pressure: 130/80 mmHg
Heart rate: 110 bpm
GCS: 14/15

Which toxicological influences can be present despite normal oxygen saturations?

Carbon monoxide and methaemoglobin can both be potentially present in significant concentrations despite normal oxygen saturations.

TIMEPOINT 2

Within 30 minutes of arrival, the emergency department doctor assigned to Mr Roberts starts working quickly because they are aware that the likely diagnosis is carbon monoxide poisoning/ car-fume inhalation and there is a need to manage Mr Roberts pro-actively. The emergency department doctor checks Mr Roberts' carboxyhaemoglobin level and finds out that the result is 17%, far above the upper limit of normal.

The team contacts the National Poisons Information Service and also speaks to the regional hyperbaric centre who advises maximal high-flow non-rebreather oxygen therapy but not hyperbaric transfer. He makes step-by-step improvements in carboxyhaemoglobin levels and oxygenation via repeated blood gas tests.

What are the clinical indicators of carbon monoxide poisoning?

There are rather few, but they may include a degree of pink/pale colouration of the lips/skin and a normal value on bedside pulse oximeter despite an appropriate history.

A physician associate student working with the acute admitting medical team sees that there is a clear need to use oxygen in Mr Roberts, but asks her colleague a question about whether every medical patient should have oxygen.

The use of oxygen for acutely admitted medical patients

Historically, innumerable numbers of acutely admitted adult medical patients, including those with a variety of cardio-respiratory disorders, arrived in emergency departments with a non-rebreather mask attached to high-flow oxygen. It is increasingly clear that oxygen is a drug that needs coordinated prescription and careful titration. Recent evidence, whilst not diminishing the need for oxygen in those for whom it is required, such as those with severe hypoxia, suggest the need for an alteration in approach.

There are now several scenarios which are linked to harm associated with unwarranted oxygen therapy. The current evidence base shows worse outcomes in patients with stroke and myocardial infarction where oxygen is not needed. New guidance now suggests not giving oxygen to those with an oxygen saturation above 93%. Patients with COPD will generally have a target saturation of 88–92%.

Similarly, alongside COPD, other patients with or at risk for Type 2 respiratory failure may have a similar target including those with some severe neuromuscular disorders, obstructive sleep apnoea, etc. As described above, higher target oxygen saturations (in the >93% category) are now generally reserved where a particular need for oxygen delivery is required, including carbon monoxide poisoning (as above), cluster headache and certain haematological emergencies such as sickle cell crisis.

When is hyperbaric oxygen indicated?

Hyperbaric oxygen is indicated when pressurised oxygen is required to increase the availability of oxygen in the body, beyond what is possible with standard oxygen delivery methods.
    It is not without risks and therefore needs to be decided upon dependent on the degree of clinical need.
    The indications for hyperbaric oxygen in carbon monoxide poisoning include:

- Carboxyhaemoglobin level > 20%
- A failure to respond to high normobaric delivery of oxygen
- Patient is a pregnant woman

In general terms, hyperbaric chambers have a range of clinical roles. Across the world there are multiple registers of hyperbaric chambers that can be single- or multi-occupancy. A general contraindication is pneumothorax. In terms of side effects, barotrauma to the ear has been reported with other adverse effects much less common. In the UK there are several regional hyperbaric centres, often associated with coastal/nautical organisations. The frequently considered indications for hyperbaric oxygen include carbon monoxide excess; decompression illness (deep sea diving–related); gas/air embolism; necrotising soft tissue infection; acute traumatic/thermic/radiation injury.

TIMEPOINT ⏱ 3

Mr Roberts is transferred with ongoing, titrated, prescribed oxygen therapy to the ward. On the medical ward, once it is felt the oxygenation issues have improved to a very significant degree, attention then turns to the factors leading to the suicide attempt. Liaison psychiatry assessment takes place, and a detailed assessment of affect, depression risk and future potential for self-harm suicidality takes place. Community-based mental health support arrangements are put in place.

Why should oxygen be prescribed as a prescription medication?

The patient safety issues related to oxygen clearly warrant the need for it to be prescribed; it is colourless, odourless and flammable. In addition, the required oxygen delivery – such as FiO_2 – for a given patient may change over time; prevention of over-oxygenation is extremely important as it is linked to lung injury and, in certain cases, hypercapnic Type 2 respiratory failure.

TIMEPOINT ⏱ 4

Four weeks later, Mr Roberts has a day with work scheduling at the lightest possible level as he scheduled a GP appointment in the morning and then a meeting with his line manager and occupational health representative in the afternoon. The meeting at the workplace involves an overall review of his physical and mental health information during his overall duration with the employer. In the second part of the meeting he is advised that professionals would join the meeting. Those joining include an employment adviser, a union member and an external occupational health adviser alongside those already present. The employer looks at:

- Areas of professional conduct and capability
- Levels of experience
- Health records

The outcome of the meeting is to calculate the Bradford Factor.

What is the Bradford Factor?

The Bradford Factor (BF) is a human resource tool that has been around for decades. It is thought to be named after work undertaken by the Bradford University School of Management. The basic idea is to find a formula that gives a numerical value to patterns of absence, with a lower score signifying a better record. It is usually used as a disciplinary tool for sickness absence – and BF use has led to people being sacked or otherwise having decisions made against them. It is a sickness absence management tool, designed to impose limits on workers' absence, not to help them overcome sickness or poor health, work-related or otherwise. It is presented as a means of dealing fairly with the employer-defined problem that many short absences are more disruptive to the employer's business activities than a single long one. The formula puts a lot of weight on individual absences, and it produces a score over a reference period, using a very simple calculation: Bradford Factor = number of unrelated absence periods^2 × days absent. For example, 10 days' absence in the reference period (a year, say) could occur as: 1 absence of 10 days, which would have a BF of $[(1 \times 1) \times 10] = 10$; 5 absences of 2 days each which would have a BF of $[(5 \times 5) \times 10] = 250$; 10 absences of 1 day each which would have a BF of $[(10 \times 10) \times 10] = 1000$.

Following the professionals' meeting, to clarify the overall outcome of recovery from the carbon monoxide episode, a neuropsychological assessment is arranged. The neuropsychological assessment demonstrates some evidence of cognitive impairment. An informal further meeting with the line manager means that the essential importance of certification of births, marriages and deaths means that Mr Roberts' work duties need to be altered. In fact, this is a collaborative outcome as Mr Roberts admits he has found thoughts of changing roles a real consideration recently. The employer finds a different role in which Mr Roberts can be deployed in an area of renewed interest, within the same organisation with no long-term salary or pension implications but incorporating some regular collective team meetings and three monthly health checks for the upcoming year. Everyone associated with Mr Roberts finds this a positive professional outcome.

The relationship between physical and mental health and the association between employees' experience at work with a range of outcomes is a topic doctors will encounter in multiple settings. It is common for doctors of various grades to be asked to provide information or maybe reports and/or liaise with employers to clarify clinical information and often work in association with the patient to ensure their professional duties are optimally matched to ensure their wellbeing.

FURTHER READING

1. www.bmj.com/content/363/bmj.k4169

Case 32

TIMEPOINT 1

Mrs Lewis is a 78-year-old retired chef, admitted for an elective anterior and posterior repair for symptomatic vaginal prolapse. She has a background of well-controlled type 2 diabetes mellitus, hypertension and generalised anxiety disorder. She takes metformin 1 g BD, sitagliptin 100 mg OD, atorvastatin 40 mg ON, amlodipine 10 mg OD, ramipril 2.5 mg OD and citalopram 10 mg OD. She is allergic to penicillin and tramadol.

Her surgery is scheduled for the early afternoon. It is uneventful, with an estimated blood loss of 400 mL. The surgeon comes to debrief her afterwards, explaining that everything went well. Mrs Lewis reports that she feels well and is keen to go home as soon as possible. The surgeon explains that it is routine to keep patients in overnight for observation, but if everything is stable and her pain is well-controlled she could go home the next day.

At 3 am, the on-call gynaecology doctor is bleeped to see Mrs Lewis as the nurses have just checked her heart rate and found it to be 130 bpm. The doctor asks the nurse to recheck Mrs Lewis' pulse manually, and the nurse confirms that she still believes it to be approximately 130 bpm.

The doctor arrives on the ward and finds Mrs Lewis sitting up in bed. She is complaining of feeling very dizzy and breathless, and has palpitations. She denies having any chest pain or discomfort.

Her observations are:

Respiratory rate: 27/min
Oxygen saturations: 96% on room air
Temperature: 36.7°C
Blood pressure: 114/87 mmHg
Heart rate: 138 bpm

The doctor examines Mrs Lewis and finds that her pulse is irregularly irregular and very fast. She is warm and well perfused peripherally with a capillary refill time of less than 2 seconds. Her cardiovascular and respiratory examination is otherwise normal, except for tachypnoea. The doctor encourages Mrs Lewis to take deep breaths and try to slow down her breathing. The doctor also checks the wound site, and there is no evidence of bleeding.

She asks the nurses to do an ECG which shows that Mrs Lewis is in atrial fibrillation with a fast ventricular rate. The doctor reviews Mrs Lewis' history with her. Mrs Lewis confirms that she has never been told that she has atrial fibrillation before. She has occasionally had chest pain on exertion in the past, but it has never lasted long, and she has never told her GP about it. She recalls having a 24-hour tape around 20 years ago, but can't remember why she had it and was told at the time that it was normal. She doesn't remember ever having an echocardiogram.

The gynaecology doctor is concerned about Mrs Lewis' fast heart rate and gives her a stat dose of 2.5 mg of bisoprolol. She then takes some blood tests while she is waiting for the bisoprolol to take effect.

What is the management of acute atrial fibrillation in a haemodynamically stable patient?

- Clarify if this is a first episode or not by discussing with the patient and checking old ECGs
- Investigate possible underlying causes. There are many things which can tip the predisposed older patient into an arrhythmia. Common causes include infection, heart

failure, electrolyte abnormalities, pulmonary embolism, anaemia and hyperthyroidism. Atrial fibrillation may spontaneously cardiovert if the underlying cause is treated

- Blood tests should be sent including full blood count, urea and electrolytes, magnesium, calcium and thyroid function tests. Other tests may be appropriate if there is a specific underlying cause suspected
- If the onset of arrhythmia has been within 48 hours, rate or rhythm control can be used. If more than 48 hours or uncertain, start rate control
- Management options include
  - Rate control
    - Beta-blocker, e.g. bisoprolol, metoprolol or carvedilol
    - Non-dihydropyridine calcium channel blockers, e.g. diltiazem or verapamil
    - Digoxin can be used in sedentary patients
  - Rhythm control
    - Chemical cardioversion with amiodarone or flecainide (flecainide should not be used in patients with evidence of structural or ischaemic heart disease)
    - Synchronised DC cardioversion if haemodynamically unstable or patient choice
- Start anticoagulation with heparin until a full assessment can be made regarding long-term anticoagulation therapy

Mrs Lewis has a chest X-ray, which is normal, to rule out pneumonia as a cause of her breathlessness. Her initial blood tests are given in Table 32.1.

Her pulse is repeated and is now around 85 bpm and regular.

The ECG is repeated and shows normal sinus rhythm with a rate of around 88 bpm.

How should patients be managed with chronic or paroxysmal atrial fibrillation?

- Rate control is usually first line
  - Beta-blocker
  - Diltiazem
  - Digoxin can be used in sedentary patients
  - If monotherapy fails, two drugs can be used in combination (monitor carefully if using diltiazem with a beta-blocker due to risk of cardiodepression)
- Rhythm control – if rate control is ineffective, or if the patient is symptomatic despite being well rate controlled
  - Pharmacological
    - Beta-blocker
    - Dronedarone to maintain sinus rhythm after cardioversion
  - 'Pill-in-the-pocket' with flecainide if paroxysmal
  - Electrical cardioversion (if in AF more than 48 hours)
    - Consider giving amiodarone for 4 weeks before and up to 12 months after to maintain sinus rhythm

Table 32.1 Venous blood results

White cell count	13.7×10^9/L	Calcium (corrected)	2.45 mmol/L
Haemoglobin	98 g/L	Albumin	44 g/L
Platelets	412×10^9/L	Bilirubin	4 µmol/L
MCV	72 fL	Alkaline phosphatase	84 U/L
Sodium	139 mmol/L	Alanine aminotransferase	26 U/L
Potassium	4.6 mmol/L	Free thyroxine (FT4)	17 pmol/L
Urea	6.1 mmol/L	Thyroid-stimulating hormone	3.1 mU/L
Creatinine	91 µmol/L	INR	1.1
C-reactive protein	54 mg/L	PT	12 secs
Troponin	Negative	APTT	43 secs
Magnesium	0.83 mmol/L	Fibrinogen	3.2 g/L

  – Patient should be anticoagulated for 3 weeks before cardioversion
- Left atrial ablation if drug treatment has failed to control symptoms
- Pacing and atrioventricular node ablation if symptomatic or with left ventricular dysfunction due to high ventricular rates
- Anticoagulation
  - Patients should also be assessed for the need for long-term anticoagulation if
    – Sinus rhythm is not restored within 48 hours
    – There is a high risk of AF recurring
    – Time of onset is unclear
  - If anticoagulation may be appropriate, calculate CHA_2DS_2-VASc and HASBLED scores. If men have a CHA_2DS_2-VASc score of 1 or higher, or any person has a CHA_2DS_2-VASc score of 2 or higher, anticoagulation with a DOAC or warfarin should be considered unless it is thought that the risk of anticoagulation outweighs the benefit

TIMEPOINT 2

The next morning, Mrs Lewis is seen on the ward round. Her heart rate settled after the dose of bisoprolol overnight, and she is now feeling much better. She asks again if she can go home today. Although there are no further gynaecological concerns, the gynaecology consultant is keen to get a cardiology opinion prior to Mrs Lewis' discharge.

After the ward round, the junior doctor on the team discusses the events of the night with the cardiology registrar and asks if there is anything that needs to be done, given that the atrial fibrillation terminated with just a small dose of bisoprolol. The cardiology registrar advises that as Mrs Lewis has a number of risk factors for the atrial fibrillation returning, it would be wise to start on her anticoagulation, as soon as the gynaecology team is happy that there is no increased postoperative bleeding risk. They also recommend repeating the ECG and requesting a non-urgent echocardiogram and 24-hour tape.

The junior doctor calculates Mrs Lewis' CHA_2DS_2-VASc score as 4, and HASBLED score as 1. He returns to Mrs Lewis after the ward round to explain that they would recommend starting anticoagulation, explaining the risks and benefits. She agrees that it sounds like a good idea, and the doctor prescribes apixaban 5 mg BD.

He asks the nursing staff to repeat the ECG. Half an hour later, the nursing staff bring the junior doctor the ECG (Figure 32.1).

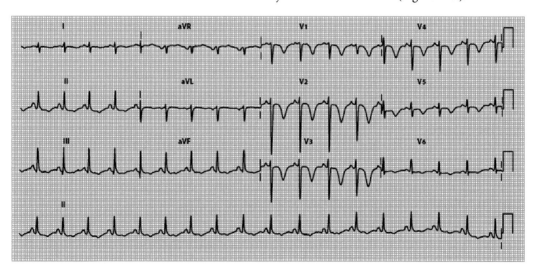

Figure 32.1 Repeat ECG. (Reproduced with permission from *Making Sense of the ECG* by Andrew R. Houghton.)

What sign is demonstrated on the ECG?

Wellens' sign or pattern.

This is where there is deep T-wave inversion in multiple precordial leads, with minimal or no ST elevation. Rarely, in a less common variant, patients may have biphasic T-waves.

What does this sign represent?

- Wellens' sign is highly suggestive of severe proximal left anterior descending coronary artery stenosis
- Patients with this sign are at extremely high risk of a major anterior myocardial infarction and death within weeks
- Patients are pain free at the time of the ECG changes
- The ECG changes are associated with a troponin that is normal or only very slightly raised (less than twice the upper limit of normal)
- Stress testing of any kind should be avoided as this could provoke an infarct
- Patients should receive urgent coronary angiography to decide if they are appropriate for stenting or CABG

Wellens' syndrome diagnostic criteria:	PLUS
• Deeply inverted and symmetrical T-waves in leads V2–V3 (sometimes also V1, V4, V5 or V6) **OR** • Biphasic T-waves in V2 and V3	• History of angina • Pain-free at the time of ECG • Troponin normal or only slightly elevated • Isoelectric or minimally elevated ST segment • No precordial Q-waves

The junior doctor bleeps the cardiology registrar to explain the ECG findings. He compares today's ECG to previous ones and confirms that Mrs Lewis has never had T-wave inversion in the past. The cardiology registrar explains that he is concerned that this could be Wellens' syndrome, and he will come to review Mrs Lewis as soon as he can.

Mrs Lewis is seen by the cardiology team who take her for an urgent angiography. The angiography shows 60% stenosis in the obtuse marginal artery. Mrs Lewis is transferred to the local cardiothoracic centre for a coronary artery bypass graft. She makes a good recovery from her surgery and is discharged directly from there, with cardiology and cardiothoracic follow-up.

TIMEPOINT 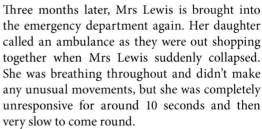 3

Three months later, Mrs Lewis is brought into the emergency department again. Her daughter called an ambulance as they were out shopping together when Mrs Lewis suddenly collapsed. She was breathing throughout and didn't make any unusual movements, but she was completely unresponsive for around 10 seconds and then very slow to come round.

She remains on atenolol, diltiazem and apixaban, as well as all the other medications she was taking when she had her first operation. When the paramedics arrived they noted that her pulse was irregularly irregular and approximately 140 bpm. Her blood pressure is 101/73 mmHg. They cannulate her and start IV fluids, and bring her in to the emergency department.

She arrives at the emergency department and is stabilised with intravenous fluids and amiodarone. Her heart rate reduces to 80 bpm, but she remains in atrial fibrillation. Her blood pressure improves to 132/89 mmHg. Mrs Lewis is otherwise well and cannot think of anything that might have precipitated her collapse. She is reviewed by the cardiology team who advise that as medical treatments have failed, they would like to offer her pacing with atrioventricular node ablation.

What are the indications for consideration of permanent pacemaker insertion?

- Prevention of atrial fibrillation and treatment of atrial fibrillation resistant to medical therapy

- Second- or third-degree atrioventricular block
- Persistent symptomatic bradycardia (sinus node disease)

When should implantable cardioverter defibrillators (ICDs) be used?

Implantable cardioverter defibrillators are devices designed to detect dangerous arrhythmias and deliver a shock to cardiovert the patient back to normal sinus rhythm.

Patients who may be appropriate include:

- Survivors of a VT or VF cardiac arrest
- Patients with sustained ventricular tachycardias
- Some patients with a previous myocardial infarction and a left ventricular ejection fraction <35%
- Patients with a condition or family history of a condition associated with sudden cardiac death, such as Brugada's syndrome and hypertrophic cardiomyopathy

Mrs Lewis has a permanent pacemaker inserted the following day, with the intention that she should undergo the ablation procedure 3 days after. The procedure goes well, and after 2 hours in the recovery bay, she is transferred up to the cardiology ward for monitoring overnight.

TIMEPOINT ⏱ 4

Two hours after her arrival on the cardiology ward, Mrs Lewis begins to feel very breathless. She complains that she is getting 'terrible pain' on her left side when she breathes in. The sister calls the junior doctor on the ward to review Mrs Lewis as she is worried that she looks as if she is working very hard to breathe and becoming tired as a result.

Her observations are:

Respiratory rate: 32/min
Oxygen saturations: 84% on room air
Temperature: 36.9°C
Blood pressure: 96/62 mmHg
Heart rate: 82 bpm

The cardiology doctor is concerned that Mrs Lewis may have sustained an iatrogenic pneumothorax during the insertion of her pacemaker. He starts Mrs Lewis on 15 litres of oxygen via a non-rebreathe mask and proceeds to examine her.

What signs might the doctor find on examination?

- Iatrogenic pneumothorax (or haemothorax) may occur after pacemaker or ICD insertion in up to 5% of cases
- This is due to the proximity of the subclavian vein, which is used for access, to the apex of the lung
- It usually develops within 48 hours of the procedure and tends to be ipsilateral
- Patients may complain of shortness of breath and pleuritic chest pain
- Signs on examination include
  - Signs of respiratory distress
  - Hypoxia
  - Cyanosis
  - Hypotension and tachycardia
  - Reduced expansion on the affected side
  - Hyper-resonance over the collapse
  - Reduced breath sounds
  - Subcutaneous emphysema

The doctor requests an urgent chest X-ray to confirm his suspicions.

What is the management of a (non-tension) pneumothorax?

- A chest X-ray should be requested to confirm the diagnosis. A pneumothorax will be seen as a visible lung edge within the lung fields, with absent lung markings peripherally
- Sometimes a lateral film is needed to see a small pneumothorax
- An ABG should be taken and oxygen given if the patient is hypoxic. Breathing oxygen also increases the speed at which the pneumothorax is resorbed
- Treatment depends on the size of the pneumothorax

- A small pneumothorax (rim of air <2 cm) is usually managed conservatively by observing to ensure that it is not increasing in size
- A larger pneumothorax may be managed using
  - Thoracocentesis (simple aspiration)
    - 21G needle inserted in the second or third intercostal space at the midclavicular line, or in the fourth or fifth intercostal space at the anterior axillary line
    - The needle should be inserted over the superior rib margin, in order to avoid the neurovascular bundle
  - Chest drain
    - More likely to be required for secondary spontaneous pneumothoraces, larger pneumothoraces, tension pneumothoraces, bilateral pneumothoraces, patients who are ventilated, or patients in which thoracocentesis has failed
  - Pleurodesis
    - This is used in patients with recurrent pneumothorax
    - Options include chemical pleurodesis with products such as talc or minocycline, or surgical pleurectomy. These may be carried out via a thoracotomy or VATS

The chest X-ray confirms a small left sided pneumothorax. The doctor attempts a thoracocentesis and repeats the X-ray, confirming resolution of the pneumothorax. The medical student on the ward asks the doctor how he knew that it wasn't a tension pneumothorax.

How can a tension pneumothorax be recognised, and how should it be managed?

- Signs of a tension pneumothorax are
  - Trachea deviated away from the side of collapse
  - Midline shift evident on the chest X-ray
  - Raised JVP
  - Severe hypotension and tachycardia (i.e. shock)
- Management
  - Give 15 litres of oxygen via a non-rebreathe mask
  - Emergency needle decompression using a large-bore (15G) needle, inserted perpendicular to the chest wall, in second or third anterior intercostal space in the mid-clavicular line
  - Leave the needle in place until the air stops leaking, then insert a definitive chest drain as soon as possible

Case 33

 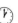
Mrs Field, aged 72, has felt generally unwell for months. She is retired, does not significantly exercise and had previously performed a sedentary occupation; it had always been suggested that she lose weight whenever at the GP. Over 3 years ago, her weight was 113 kg, height 1.65 m and BMI 41.5.

At that time an HbA1c test was 45 mmol/mol and the GP, when describing the result, had said something about risk of diabetes and a possible national diabetes prevention programme.

More recently, she has become increasingly concerned about her chances of developing health problems because a friend of hers who bought the same dress size had recently been diagnosed with diabetes. Her mother had 'gone blind' from diabetes, and that also was a concern.

Nonetheless, since she became a widow 4 years ago, her lack of activity had been combined with just 'eating to feel better' in connection with the sadness of her loss and loneliness. Before the day of admission, she had last been seen by her closest friend over a month ago, because they'd postponed a couple of their usual coffee mornings. She did have regular telephone contact with her son who lived in Australia, and she told him she was feeling gradually less well over the last few months. He normally came over to the UK around once a year, but upon hearing that his mother had been really unwell, he flew over, went straight from the airport and was shocked by the sight of seeing his mother lying down quite drowsy on the sofa and immediately called an ambulance.

The paramedics arrived and found that Mrs Field was only responding to pain on the AVPU scale. They did a glucose fingerprick reading, and the answer was unrecordably 'HIGH'.

What might give a falsely inaccurate fingerprick glucose reading?

The finger itself needs to be clean, dry and free of any alcohol-based cleaning fluid or any preceding contact with high sugar-content products such as honey, jam or fruit; in addition the drop of blood needs to be sufficient, on a test strip that is not beyond its expiration date and has been stored at the appropriate temperature. The rest of her observations shows:

Respiratory rate: 24/min
Oxygen saturations: 95% on room air
Temperature: 36.5°C
Blood pressure: 115/70 mmHg
Heart rate: 86 bpm

The paramedics decide to rush her via pre-alert to the nearest emergency department.

TIMEPOINT 2

Ten minutes later, in the emergency department, the ECG shows non-specific T-wave changes, sinus rhythm and nil else of note. The emergency department nurse asks for rapid assessment by a senior doctor and, having received paramedic handover, they start intravenous fluids and send urgent blood tests to the laboratory.

Laboratory blood results are called through:

Venous blood results

Sodium	156 mmol/L
Potassium	4.5 mmol/L
Urea	41 mmol/L
Glucose	43 mmol/L
Ketones	0.4 µmol/L

The calculated osmolality is 340 mosmol/kg.

The team decides that the most likely diagnosis is hyperglycaemic hyperosmolar state (HHS) and immediately call the duty medical team.

Why is HHS linked with such severe morbidity and mortality?

The mechanism behind this condition is multimodal and involves the fact that sufficient insulin is present (in most cases) to avoid severe ketosis/diabetic ketoacidosis; however, the osmotic effect of the hyperglycaemia brings about severe dehydration coupled with the fact that many patients are elderly with reduced renal reserve. Increased pro-inflammatory cytokines may be part of the process leading to higher risk of cardiovascular and thrombotic complications. Despite all the above, the signficantly higher mortality of HHS compared to DKA still needs further study.

TIMEPOINT 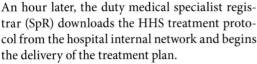 3

An hour later, the duty medical specialist registrar (SpR) downloads the HHS treatment protocol from the hospital internal network and begins the delivery of the treatment plan.

The medical SpR is working alongside a medical student who asks what the major points to look out for might be in managing HHS. She describes how the key issues in managing HHS are meticulous management of fluid balance, given the acute kidney injury/raised creatinine often present, and potential alteration in cardiac function and avoidance of hypoglycaemia due to over-provision of insulin. The UK guidelines

suggest very strict criteria for the initiation of intravenous insulin in this condition, and then only at a rate of 0.05 units/kg/hour.

Mrs Field appears relatively stable as the treatment with intravenous fluid continues.

Her repeat observations are:

Respiratory rate: 18/min
Oxygen saturations: 95% on room air
Temperature: 36°C
Blood pressure: 115/70 mmHg
Heart rate: 80 bpm

Repeat blood tests 6 hours after admission show:

Venous blood results

Sodium	157 mmol/L
Potassium	4.3 mmol/L
Urea	22 mmol/L
Glucose	19.7 µmol/L

A student nurse is given feedback because the incorrect bed and equipment were brought for Mrs Field whilst she was being transferred to the ward. As part of her self-directed learning, she decides to learn more about the needs of bariatric patients in healthcare.

What are some of the needs of bariatric patients in healthcare settings?

Internationally, more and more people are overweight or obese, meaning that in healthcare settings, the needs of the bariatric patient are becoming more important. Varied definitions are given for a bariatric patient; options include BMI ≥35 with comorbidities, BMI ≥40 or weight ≥150 kg.

A range of organisations have brought out guidelines for such patients, including the Society for Obesity and Bariatric Anaesthesia. Issues to consider include the safe transfer of patients to and from the health facility, and enabling appropriate seating/trolley/bedding equipment. From a healthcare worker point of view, lifting and handling issues mean a need for greater education and bespoke equipment. This is linked with 'risk assessments' that need to incorporate accurate height, weight, BMI and similar measurements of the patient. The bariatric patient may require weight-adjusted prophylactic medication against venous thromboembolism, may have the need for increased pressure area vigilance and might need medication doses adjusted to account for lean body weight in comparison to total body weight.

TIMEPOINT ⏱ 4

On the ward, throughout the following morning, ongoing observations are performed and show a gradual slight fall in pulse and rise in blood pressure.

The nurses provide assistance around the bedside whilst doing their morning medication round; it is clear that Mrs Field is feeling somewhat better and sits in the ward bed with the opportunity to read a favourite novel. Her concerns and questions for the healthcare team centre around how she might manage the diabetes after discharge. The ward nurse calls the diabetes inpatient specialist nurse (DISN), who, with use of a proforma, completes a full assessment and management plan for Mrs Field including telephone support after leaving the hospital.

Venous blood results

Sodium	145 mmol/L
Potassium	4.1 mmol/L
Urea	22 mmol/L
Glucose	134 µmol/L

> It is notable that the sodium level has improved but an elevated creatinine remains. Some people post-HHS are left with incomplete recovery of renal function post-AKI.

Hypernatremia

Mrs Field had hypernatremia. It is an elevated sodium level >145 mmol/L. The causes are varied and importantly, the management is completely different dependent on the cause. It can be associated with an osmotic factor and effective dehydration such as in the process leading to HHS. It is very important to distinguish between HHS and diabetes insipidus (DI), because the treatment needs to be entirely different, and in severe cases of DI, the patient may urgently need desmopressin therapy. Investigations may include levels of serum glucose, calcium, urate, serum osmolality and paired urine sodium and osmolality. When treating, a gradual fall in the sodium level is recommended.

What is the role for inpatient diabetes teams?

In hospitals around the world, the prevalence of diabetes in inpatients is higher than the general population and is often 15–20%. That is partly because many patients with diabetic foot issues and other major cardiovascular conditions such as cardiac and renal disease have a high prevalence inside hospitals. Data gathered across many settings demonstrate that diabetes inpatient specialist nurses are key to high-quality care. They have multiple roles, including consultations with patients, but also staff education, awareness of patient safety issues, work with consultants/attending specialists in diabetes and performing a wide liaison role with community diabetes professionals.

Mrs Field leaves the hospital on a twice-daily 'biphasic insulin' on discharge; she will have telephone and face-to-face follow-up and data are entered onto a diabetes database. She is also given an information sheet and access to a relevant website that details the expected range of annual checks that should take place.

Can diabetes be prevented?

All governments are interested in reducing the rate of increase in cases of type 2 diabetes, and concerted efforts to develop an evidence base for this have taken place. Randomised diabetes prevention intervention studies have most recently looked at various diet and exercise regimes, including enhancements such as dietetic and/or personal trainer 'coaching'. In the UK, a selective specially designed diabetes prevention programme (DPP) is up and running.

The entry criteria are people with fasting glucose 5.5–6.9 mmol/L and/or an HbA1c of 42–47 mmol/mol. In other words, these are people 'just below' the glycaemic criteria for diabetes.

The core components of the programme include reducing weight, altering diet and increasing activity. The programme includes multiple sessions over a minimum 9-month period, involving extensive face-to-face contact and goal-setting support.

Alongside all of this, government subsidies and/or economic support have tried to enable referrals for well-recognised weight loss companies, which has improved access.

Finally, there is much interest in very low-calorie diets (VLCD), e.g. 800 calories per day, with published data suggesting benefit – in certain people – in that some people do see remission of 'diabetes' status from a glycaemic point of view; again, this is being tried as another form of intervention.

FURTHER READING

1. https://abcd.care/sites/abcd.care/files/
resources/JBDS_IP_HHS_Adults.pdf

Case 34

Mr Nok, a 63-year-old recently retired bank clerk, goes to see his GP due to progressive tiredness, achy joints and gradual weight gain. His wife was surprised by how his activities had slowed in those months, contrary to the extra energy she expected him to have upon retirement from a long and conscientious career. They are from an Afro-Caribbean background.

Mr Nok is referred by his primary-care doctor to the acute internal medicine ambulatory care clinic, due to the finding of an unexplained calcium level of 3.01 mmol/L on a set of blood tests.

On arrival at the ambulatory care clinic, a history is taken that reveals non-specific tiredness over months, and a feeling of a slight change in body shape with an increase in waist size and maybe reduced muscle bulk. Mr Nok looks somewhat tired but not acutely unwell.

His observations show:

Respiratory rate: 18/min
Oxygen saturations: 95% on room air
Temperature: 37°C
Blood pressure: 148/82 mmHg
Heart rate: 81 bpm

Examination demonstrates a height of 1.8 m, weight of 100 kg and BMI of 30.86.

He has relatively sparse axillary and pubic hair and the testicular size is found to be around 6 mL bilaterally. Mr Nok wonders what that means and is keen for tests to take place to understand the clinical findings. The doctor who examined him says that nothing specific on examination suggests a particular cause for the raised calcium and further tests would be done.

What are the key aspects in assessing testicular size?

Testicular size is relevant in any case where pubertal progress is important and/or a condition that may affect gonadotropin/androgen status. It is done by both inspection and palpation, and, whilst expecting a slight degree of asymmetry, one should find bilateral testes with volumes appropriate for age. The normal volumetric status for an adult male is approximately 20–25 mL. There are age-appropriate scales available for testicular volume linked with pubertal stage of development. The volume can be accurately assessed using equipment called an orchidometer.

Further blood tests and a chest X-ray are performed to investigate the testicular finding and the hypercalcaemia; they take place the next morning in the fasting state – results show:

Venous blood results

FSH [1–7 IU/L]	0.3 IU/L
LH [1–8 IU/L]	0.4 IU/L
Testosterone [6.7–31 nmol/L]	5.7 nmol/L
Prolactin [<700 mIU/L]	367 mIU/L
Cortisol [>350 nmol/L]	359 nmol/L
TSH [0.4–4.5 mU/L]	1.2 mU/L
T4 [12–22 pmol/L]	12.7 pmol/L
ACE [8–52 u/L]	45 u/L
PTH [1.6–6.9 pmol/L]	2.1 pmol/L
Vitamin D [>50 nmol/L]	51 nmol/L
Calcium	2.9 mmol/L
Fasting glucose	5.7 mmol/L
Creatinine	116 µmol/L

Table 34.1 Differential diagnoses of hypercalcaemia

Hypercalcaemia with normal or raised PTH	Hypercalcaemia with low PTH
Primary hyperparathyroidism	Malignancy – solid tumours/Parathyroid hormone-related protein effect
Parathyroid carcinoma	Myeloma
Familial hypocalciuric hypercalcaemia	Sarcoidosis/other causes of excess vitamin D

TIMEPOINT ⏱ 2

Two days later, on a visit back to the ambulatory care clinic, the results of the wider panel of blood tests are discussed. The internal medicine doctor seeing Mr Nok is unsure how to interpret the results but is puzzled that the parathyroid hormone level is below the reference range alongside a raised calcium and so asks his senior colleague. In addition, the report of the chest X-ray has returned. Chest X-ray report: *clear lung fields and bilateral hilar lymph node prominence.*

What are the causes of hypercalcaemia, and how does the PTH level differ in those various scenarios?

Table 34.1 mentions a few of the more important common differentials of hypercalcaemia.

Mr Nok is informed that sarcoidosis is the most likely condition to explain the results obtained thus far; referrals are made to the appropriate specialist services – those include the rheumatology (subspecialist sarcoidosis) clinic and the endocrinology clinic to look into the testicular/testosterone status.

TIMEPOINT ⏱ 3

A month later, Mr Nok comes to see the specialist at the rheumatology centre. Treatment for sarcoidosis in the form of oral prednisolone 40 mg is commenced. Mr Nok reveals more history in that alongside the somewhat unexpected weight gain of 8 kg over 6 months, he has felt a bit 'muzzy headed' with occasional headaches, and it happens to be that the doctor seeing Mr Nok had previously worked with a neurologist with a special interest in neurosarcoidosis.

An MRI scan of the brain is done – it shows some altered signal around the hypothalamus and given the probable presence of a systemic condition such as sarcoid, it is suggested that neurosarcoidosis is a possible interpretation. Mr Nok then undergoes a neurological evaluation and is booked into the neurosarcoid clinic.

What are some of the key organ-based manifestations of sarcoidosis?

Sarcoidosis is a multisystem granulomatous condition associated with hypercalcaemia and a variety of end-organ manifestations.

- Skin: lupus pernio, erythema nodosum
- Cardiovascular system: conduction defects
- Central nervous system: neurosarcoid, cranial nerve defects
- Musculoskeletal system: joint pain
- Eyes: uveitis, nodules, glaucoma, cataracts
- Lungs: lymph node enlargement, pulmonary nodules

TIMEPOINT ⏱ 4

Two months later, Mr Nok returns to the combined rheumatology/neurology neurosarcoidosis clinic and on the same afternoon he is conveniently able to attend the endocrinology clinic.

It is concluded that appetite alteration caused by a central effect of the neurosarcoid involvement of the hypothalamus is the clinical process taking place.

Evaluation demonstrates that 6 kg weight loss has taken place.

As his disease is now stable, it is felt that the balance of benefit against risk favours tapering his prednisolone downwards, so it is agreed to start tapering the prednisolone.

At the endocrinology clinic the following questions arise from a medical student attending outpatients.

The level of testosterone has been shown to be low; what level is low enough to initiate testosterone treatment?

The international guidelines on this topic suggest initiating testosterone if total fasting morning values are <8 nmol/L or if there is a low bio-available testosterone in the presence of suitable symptoms.

What types of testosterone treatments are available?

The preparations of testosterone include oral tablets, transdermal gels and injectable forms. The oral tablets are subject to first-pass metabolism and have not been found to have favourable or predictable clinical effects, and thus, are not commonly used. Several transdermal gel formulations are frequently prescribed; they have a dose range that can be suited to clinical need and are locally administered on a daily basis, usually on the upper arms, with precautions to optimise absorption and reduce risk of contact with other people whilst the gel is still present on the skin. Finally, another commonly prescribed type of testosterone treatment is an injectable form, either lasting 2–3 weeks, or more frequently a depot formulation – these are given intramuscularly every 10–12 weeks.

Is it a recognised phenomenon to see reproductive system alteration in sarcoidosis?

Sarcoidosis may affect individuals of reproductive age and can affect the patient in a wide variety of ways.

Neurosarcoidosis affecting the hypothalamus and/or pituitary can lead to altered prolactin and/or reduced LH or FSH. Additionally, changes in TRH/TSH may lead to variable thyroid function. In men, testicular involvement can cause inflammation and/or changes in testosterone production/spermatogenesis. In women, uterine involvement and/or granulomatous disease in the ovaries/fallopian tubes may lead to menstrual alteration. Comprehensive evaluation is needed with regard to aspects of fertility and pregnancy.

Case 35

Mrs Brown, a 63-year-old librarian, attends her GP with a 3-day history of headache. Although she is known to suffer from migraine with aura, she denies any visual symptoms and says that this is 'not like her usual headache'. Her current headache is mostly at the sides of her head, with a severity of 7/10. The pain is equal on both sides.

She also complains of feeling tired and generally unwell. She has aches and pains 'all over', but her shoulders are particularly bothering her.

On examination, her observations are:

Respiratory rate: 18/min
Oxygen saturations: 97% on room air
Temperature: 37.4°C
Blood pressure: 137/86 mmHg

Heart rate: 73 bpm

Her GCS is 15, and she has an entirely normal cranial nerve, upper limb and lower limb neurological examination. She has no neck stiffness.

Mrs Brown has a past medical history of asthma, for which she takes a regular steroid inhaler and PRN salbutamol. She does not have any drug allergies. She lives with her husband and two cats. She enjoys the occasional glass of wine with dinner and stopped smoking socially in her 30s.

What are the key features that help you to narrow down your differential diagnosis for a presenting complaint of 'headache'?

See Figure 35.1.

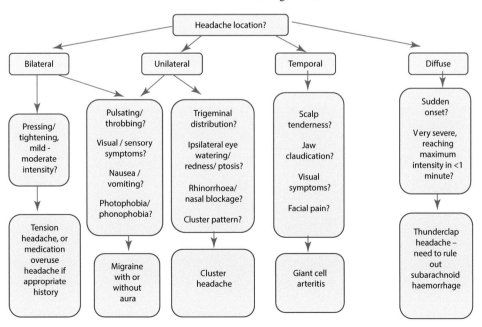

Figure 35.1 Differential diagnosis of headache.

DOI: 10.1201/9781351257725-35

According to NICE guidelines, what are the 'red flag' headache features which warrant further investigation or referral?

- Worsening headache with fever
- Sudden onset headache, reaching maximum intensity within 5 minutes
- New onset neurological deficit
- New onset cognitive dysfunction
- Personality change
- Impaired level of consciousness
- Head trauma within 3 months
- Headache triggered by cough, valsalva, sneeze, exercise or changes in posture
- Headache with symptoms suggestive of giant cell arteritis
- Headache with symptoms suggestive of acute narrow angle glaucoma
- Existing headache with a substantial change in characteristics
- New onset headache in immunocompromised patient
- New onset headache in patient under 20 years with a history of malignancy
- New onset headache in a patient with a history of malignancy known to metastasise to the brain
- Vomiting in a patient with no obvious cause

The GP decides to send some blood tests but is reassured by the absence of any red flag symptoms. Mrs Brown is discharged with a prescription for codeine and a diagnosis of likely tension-type headache.

TIMEPOINT ⏱ 2

Two days later, Mrs Brown presents to her local emergency department complaining of blurred vision. She was driven in by her husband as she was worried that it would not be safe for her to drive. Her headache and joint pains that she told the GP about are still ongoing and she still does not quite feel herself. She is now also reporting pain when chewing, which has been coming on towards the end of her meals.

Her observations are:

Respiratory rate: 16/min
Oxygen saturations: 96% on room air
Temperature: 38.2°C
Blood pressure: 136/85 mmHg
Heart rate: 77 bpm

Systems examination is unremarkable except for tenderness over the left temple.

Visual examination demonstrates normal eye movements and reflexes. Uncorrected acuity is 6/60 in the left eye, and 6/12 in the right eye. The left eye has a central field defect. Fundoscopy demonstrates a healthy-appearing right retina. On the left side, there is oedema of the optic disc with adjacent retinal whitening and cotton wool spots.

The emergency department doctor checks the blood tests sent by the GP 2 days prior.

Her blood tests are given in Table 35.1.

Given the combination of headache, blurred vision and a raised ESR, the emergency department doctor is concerned about the possibility

Table 35.1 Venous blood results

White cell count	21.1×10^9/L	Urea	5.3 mmol/L
Haemoglobin	96 g/L	Creatinine	76 µmol/L
Platelets	586×10^9/L	Albumin	48 g/L
MCV	82 fL	Bilirubin	11 µmol/L
Sodium	139 mmol/L	Alkaline phosphatase	152 U/L
Potassium	4.6 mmol/L	Alanine aminotransferase	29 U/L
C-reactive protein	74 mg/L	ESR	93 mm/hr

of giant cell arteritis (temporal arteritis). He also notes that she is describing what sounds like jaw claudication, and the joint symptoms she relates may reflect undiagnosed polymyalgia rheumatica.

What are the American College of Rheumatology diagnostic criteria for giant cell arteritis?

American College of Rheumatology criteria (three out of five needed):

- Onset at age ≥50 years
- New onset headache
- Temporal artery tenderness to palpation or decreased pulsation
- ESR ≥50 mm/hour
- Abnormal artery biopsy, showing vasculitis characterised by a predominance of mononuclear cell infiltration or granulomatous inflammation, usually with multinucleated giant cells

As Mrs Brown fits the diagnostic criteria, she is started on steroids and aspirin 75 mg daily. She is also referred for a temporal artery biopsy.

What would be an appropriate initial course of steroids? How could this be weaned?

- 60 mg prednisolone daily for 4 weeks, followed by a weaning dose
- It can take up to 2 years to wean down prednisolone safely
- Suggested weaning regime according to the British Society of Rheumatology
  - Continue 40–60 mg daily until symptoms and laboratory abnormalities resolve
  - Reduce the dose by 10 mg every 2 weeks to 20 mg
  - Then reduce by 2.5 mg every 2–4 weeks to 10 mg
  - Then reduce by 1 mg every 1–2 months, provided there is no relapse

A sample prednisolone weaning regime is given in Table 35.2.

Temporal artery biopsy confirms the diagnosis of giant cell arteritis. Mrs Brown's symptoms start to improve, and she is discharged after 1 week with a course of steroids to complete.

TIMEPOINT 3

Two weeks later, Mrs Brown is brought to A&E again by her husband. He reports that over the last couple of days she has been acting increasingly strangely. She has started refusing to let him cook for her, when usually he cooks dinner most nights. He also thinks that she has become more forgetful recently. The emergency department doctor asks Mrs Brown if there is anything that she is worried about. Mrs Brown asks that her husband leave the cubicle, before explaining that she has realised that he is a spy and that she is being tracked by MI6. She knows this because her phone line has been tampered with, and there is a van outside their house which is watching her. She will not let her husband cook for her anymore in case he attempts to poison her.

The emergency department doctor reassures Mrs Brown that he understands her concerns, and documents a mental state examination.

What are the components of the mental state examination?

- Appearance
  - Are there any distinctive features of the patient's appearance?
  - Is there evidence of self-harm?
  - Is their clothing appropriate for the season and occasion?
  - Is their personal hygiene acceptable?
- Behaviour
  - Any aspects of non-verbal communication, including body language, eye contact, facial expressions, level of arousal and general rapport
- Mood
  - How the patient reports that they feel, e.g. low, anxious, elated
- Affect
  - Observation of the patient's mood, e.g. euphoric, sad, agitated, flat, labile

Table 35.2 Sample prednisolone weaning regime

Week	Daily dose	Week	Daily dose	Week	Daily dose
1–4	60 mg	19–22	15 mg	59–66	6 mg
5–6	50 mg	23–26	12.5 mg	67–74	5 mg
7–8	40 mg	27–34	10 mg	75–82	4 mg
9–10	30 mg	35–42	9 mg	83–90	3 mg
11–14	20 mg	43–50	8 mg	91–98	2 mg
15–18	17.5 mg	51–58	7 mg	99–106	1 mg

- Speech
  - Rate of speech – excessively slow or fast?
  - Tone of speech – monotonous? Tremulous?
  - Volume of speech – quiet? Loud?
  - Quantity of speech – excessive? Minimal? Absent?
  - Fluency – articulate? Slurred?
- Cognition
  - Deficit in memory, attention, concentration or orientation?
- Thought
  - Speed – excessively slow or fast?
  - Coherence and flow – linear? Circumstantial? Tangential? Perseveration? Incoherent?
  - Content – suicidal thoughts, obsessions, overvalued ideas
  - Possession – insertion, withdrawal or broadcasting?
- Perception
  - Hallucinations?
- Insight
  - Does that patient understand that they have a problem or that what they are experiencing is abnormal?

The emergency department doctor is concerned about Mrs Brown's mental state and asks the acute psychiatric team to attend to review her. They believe that the steroid treatment Mrs Brown is receiving has induced an acutely psychotic state. As they are unable to reduce her steroid dose, they start her on 10 mg of olanzapine and admit her to the acute psychiatric ward for further observation.

Why are second-generation (atypical) antipsychotics preferred to first-generation (typical) antipsychotics?

Second-generation (atypical) antipsychotics, such as olanzapine, risperidone and quetiapine, are generally preferred as they are less likely to cause extra-pyramidal side effects. These include:

- Acute dystonia – involuntary muscle contractions. May include oculogyric crisis and torticollis
- Parkinsonism – resting tremor, bradykinesia, shuffling gait, cogwheel rigidity, mask-like facies
- Akathisia – urge to move or restlessness, usually of the lower limbs
- Tardive dyskinesia – causes a combination of involuntary slow writhing and sudden jerking movements

TIMEPOINT ⏱ 4

Ten years later, Mrs Brown, now aged 73, is being visited by her son and his family. She is carrying in a tray of tea and biscuits from the kitchen when she trips over her cat and falls onto her left side. She is unable to get up again or move her left leg. Her son calls for an ambulance, and she is taken to the emergency department.

She is clearly in a lot of pain despite paracetamol and a small dose of morphine. Observations are normal. On examination she is unable to weight bear and will not allow the doctor to move her leg passively at all. Her left leg appears externally rotated and shortened compared to the right. On the right side she has a good range of active and passive movement.

What risk factors does Mrs Brown have for osteoporosis?

- Age
- Female gender
- Prolonged high-dose steroid use
- Other risk factors which could be enquired about include: family history, past medical history of fragility fracture, smoking, low BMI, alcohol use and premature menopause

A plain AP pelvic film and lateral film of the left hip joint are done. See Figures 35.2 and 35.3.

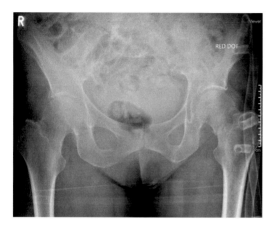

Figure 35.2 Pelvic radiograph showing a minimally displaced intracapsular left femoral neck fracture.

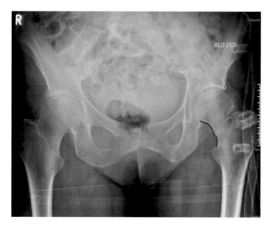

Figure 35.3 Same radiograph with red outline indicating cortical discontinuity and blue outline indicating the lucency of the fracture.

The orthopaedic team attend to review Mrs Brown. They explain that the type of hip fracture she has had means that she will need a total hip replacement. Mrs Brown goes for surgery the next day. She recovers well from her surgery, remaining an inpatient on the orthogeriatric ward for 2 weeks for further rehabilitation. She mentions to the physiotherapist that she is planning to complain about her GP, as she was told by the ward doctors that her fracture was due to osteoporosis which the GP should have assessed and treated her for.

In which patients should fracture risk be assessed, and how?

- Fracture risk should be assessed in all women aged 65 years and over, and all men aged 75 years and over
- Fracture risk should be measured in younger patients with an additional risk factor such as
  - Previous fragility fracture
  - Current or frequent recent use of oral or systemic glucocorticoids
  - History of falls
  - Family history of hip fracture
  - Other causes of secondary osteoporosis
  - Low body mass index
  - Smoking
  - Alcohol intake ≥14 units per week for women or ≥21 units per week for men
- Use FRAX or QFracture scores to estimate the patient's 10-year fracture risk (QFracture is based on UK data). FRAX is preferable if a bone mineral density (BMD) score is available
- Primary prevention management
  - Low risk
    - Lifestyle advice
      - Good nutrition
      - Exercise
      - Smoking and alcohol cessation
    - Measures to reduce falls
      - Reduction of polypharmacy
    - Calcium and vitamin D supplementation if needed
  - Intermediate risk – arrange a DXA scan to check bone mineral density and then recalculate the FRAX score

- High risk
  - As per low risk, plus
    - Bisphosphonates
      - Alendronate is usually first line
      - Risedronate or etidronate may be required in patients if alendronate is not an option and they have certain risk factors
  - If no bisphosphonates are suitable, denosumab or strontium may be used
  - Raloxifene is not recommended for primary prevention but may sometimes be used in secondary prevention

Bone mineral density categories	
T scores	standard deviations compared to a young healthy population
Z scores	compared to cohort of same age
Normal	hip BMD T score ≥–1 (i.e. 1 standard deviation below the young healthy population mean)
Osteopenia	hip BMD T score –1 to –2.5
Osteoporosis	hip BMD T score ≤–2.5
Severe osteoporosis	hip BMD T score ≤–2.5 plus a fragility fracture

FURTHER READING

1. BSP and BHPR guidelines for the management of giant cell arteritis: https://academic.oup.com/rheumatology/article/49/8/1594/1789465
2. NICE CG24 – Hip fracture management: https://www.nice.org.uk/guidance/cg124/chapter/Recommendations
3. NICE CG146 – Osteoporosis, assessing the risk of fragility fracture: https://www.nice.org.uk/guidance/cg146
4. NICE CG150 – Headaches in over 12s, diagnosis and management: https://www.nice.org.uk/guidance/cg150/chapter/Recommendations
5. Psychiatric Adverse Effects of Corticosteroids (Thomas P Warrington, J.Michael Bostwick): https://www.mayoclinicproceedings.org/article/S0025-6196(11)61160-9/pdf

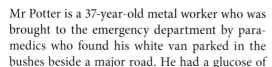

Case 36

Mr Potter is a 37-year-old metal worker who was brought to the emergency department by paramedics who found his white van parked in the bushes beside a major road. He had a glucose of 1.4 mmol/L when they tested it.

He was given emergency glucose treatment, and a partial response to the hypoglycaemia took place before arrival at hospital.

That day, he had been driving his van from one of his company's offices to another. The previous night had been his brother's 40th birthday which was spent in the local pub.

He had a 28-year history of type 1 diabetes and had not attended the diabetes clinic at the hospital for the last 6 years due to moving house, letters being directed to the wrong address, changes in relationship and other reasons. He uses NovoRapid with meals for his diabetes and Lantus once per day.

He is admitted for overnight observation of glucose and inpatient diabetes review.

On arrival at the emergency department, his observations are:

Respiratory rate: 16/min
Oxygen saturations: 99% on room air
Temperature: 36.6°C
Blood pressure: 127/80 mmHg
Heart rate: 91 bpm

In terms of alertness, Mr Potter is 'V' on the AVPU scale, responding to voice. Fingertips have visible evidence of blood testing, and in the abdomen, two egg-sized areas of firm but mobile prominent subcutaneous tissue are noticeable.

Medical aspects of fitness to drive

Many health conditions may affect a patient's ability to drive, either temporarily or in the long term. In the UK, this is regulated by the DVLA, and their website has detailed information categorising which conditions they need to be informed about.

There is no doubt that impaired hypoglycaemic awareness and the safety of driving are a significant issue; vigilance about and assessment of hypoglycaemia risk from insulin secretagogue oral therapy and all forms of insulin therapy are broadly regarded as an essential aspect of diabetes care.

Which blood tests should be considered at this point?

- FBC
- U&Es
- LFTs
- HbA1c
- Tissue transglutaminase
- Cortisol and adrenal antibodies
- TFTs and thyroid antibodies
- Lipid profile

What is the differential diagnosis of hypoglycaemia?

In people with diabetes on treatment, the most common associated medications are

DOI: 10.1201/9781351257725-36

sulphonylureas, insulin secretagogues and insulin. Away from diabetes, liver failure, adrenal insufficiency, coeliac disease, insulinoma, non-insulinoma pancreatogenous hypoglycaemia (NIPH) and glycogen storage disease are important differentials.

TIMEPOINT ⏱ 2

The next morning, Mr Potter is seen by a diabetes nurse, who goes through a range of educational aspects. She runs through an 'inpatient diabetes' proforma which looks towards a care plan for each patient and enquires about the annual 'key checks' everyone with diabetes should have each year. She interprets the prominent areas either side of the umbilicus as areas of lipohypertrophy signifying recurrent insulin injection into the same site.

Therefore, her recommendations include rotating injection sites, maintaining telephone contact, arranging a specialist clinic appointment and setting up attendance at a 5-day structured education course. She assesses hypoglycaemic awareness using the 'Clarke score'. Before discharge she also firmly encourages Mr Potter to immediately phone both the DVLA and his employer in relation to the issue of driving.

What is impaired hypoglycaemic awareness, and how can it be improved?

Impaired hypoglycaemic awareness is the reduced ability to sense the signs of glucose levels falling well below the normal range; it is a factor in the risks of adverse outcomes especially if severe enough that the lack of awareness leads to the need for other people (third parties) to intervene to treat the low glucose.

It represents both an inability for counter-regulatory systems to ensure relatively rapid falls in glucose to not take place, alongside a reduced detection/symptomatic mechanism for the person to be aware it is happening.

In the UK, NICE guidance (and similar advice internationally) suggests using either a 'Clarke' or 'Gold' score, which have several self-reported elements to 'score' awareness.

Evidence suggests that attention to various methods of optimising glycaemic control/variability can improve awareness, several of which include newer basal insulin options, accredited structured education (e.g. DAFNE), new technologies – e.g. continuous subcutaneous insulin infusions (CSII) and continuous glucose monitoring (CGM).

TIMEPOINT ⏱ 3

Around 4 months later, Mr Potter has maintained regular telephone interaction with his diabetes specialist nurse and has attended a diabetes specialist clinic to meet a consultant. Liaison with his employer's occupational health service means that adapted duties are arranged for a 6-month period whilst these key diabetes-related interventions take place. After making appropriate arrangements, he is scheduled for, takes annual leave and attends a 5-day structured type 1 diabetes education course known as the 'Dose Adjustment for Normal Eating' (DAFNE) course. A major trial published in the BMJ showed benefits of this peer-connecting professionally delivered course, and it is now seen as a core step towards improved glycaemic control in type 1 diabetes; versions of it are delivered across the world, and extremely positive feedback is usually provided by those patients who attend.

What are some of the new technologies for improving glycaemia in type 1 diabetes?

Around the world, highly motivated people are involved with type 1 diabetes research, and a race is on to harness the available and emerging technologies to improve variability in glucose levels that so many people experience. In the UK, a combination of sequential NICE guidance and a recent statement from Diabetes UK places three initial technological options at the forefront of decision-making – assuming the patient has done an accredited carbohydrate-counting course and has optimised frequent blood glucose monitoring. The key technologies incorporate three core systems, two of which are monitors – flash monitoring (such as Freestyle Libre™), continuous monitoring and the one insulin-delivery system known as an insulin pump.

There is high-quality randomised controlled and longitudinal clinical data regarding the use of insulin pump therapy (which only contains quick-acting insulin, dispensing with the need for a long-acting basal insulin). There is a range of evidence, including systematic reviews, that demonstrate the clinical benefits of both insulin pump systems and/or continuous glucose monitors. Highly specialised diabetes teams work with the patient to identify the best option given each individual patient's particular circumstances. People sometimes use combinations of these options, and newer 'smart-pumps' increasingly can recognise and act on a monitor that detects certain levels or changes in glucose and adjust insulin delivery – a fully automated system that delivers this has been called the 'closed loop'.

TIMEPOINT ⏱ 4

Approximately 8 months later, Mr Potter is now back to his previous job role, having had clearance to do so via his company's occupational health, line manager and the DVLA. He has very much better hypoglycaemic awareness and is much more confident about his diabetes. He now uses a different insulin regime and avoids all the previous injection areas. He still finds the regular glucose checks and need for constant 'glycaemic attentiveness' a challenge but has adapted to it, and is broadly positive about his improved situation.

What are the most common insulins used in type 1 diabetes?

In those patients treated with meal-time (bolus) insulin separate to a basal (background) insulin, i.e. the basal–bolus system, most commonly patients use the following:

For bolus insulins: NovoRapid, Humalog and Fiasp.
For basal insulins: Levemir (Detemir), Lantus (Glargine) or Tresiba (Degludec).

FURTHER READING

1. https://assets.publishing.service.gov.uk/government/uploads/system/uploads/attachmentdata/file/670819/assessing-fitness-to-drive-a-guide-for-medical-professionals.pdf
2. www.nice.org.uk/guidance/ng17/chapter/1-Recommendations#education-and-information-2

Case 37

TIMEPOINT 1

Mrs Atkins is a 93-year-old woman who has been admitted to hospital following a fall at home. She got out of bed in the night to go to the bathroom, had felt dizzy and ended up on the floor, unable to get herself back up again. She doesn't think she hit her head or lost consciousness. She used her pendant alarm to call for help.

Her past medical history includes type 2 diabetes mellitus, hypertension, atrial fibrillation (on apixaban), bilateral total hip replacements, previous cataract surgery, previous myocardial infarction and hypothyroidism.

She lives alone in a bungalow following the death of her husband a year ago. She has no carers, but family live locally and help with her shopping. She mobilises around the house with a frame.

Her observations are:

Respiratory rate: 22/min
Oxygen saturations: 95% on room air
Temperature: 36.8°C
Blood pressure: 102/65 mmHg
Heart rate: 72 bpm

On auscultation of her chest, there are crackles at the right base. Heart sounds are normal. She appears confused with an AMTS of 6/10. Neurological examination is normal with no external evidence of head injury. Abdominal examination is unremarkable. Chronic venous eczema is present in the lower limbs bilaterally with mild pitting oedema to the ankles.

What investigations would be appropriate to arrange?

- Bloods – FBC, U&Es, LFTs, CRP, glucose, TFTs, B12, folate, ferritin
- Chest X-ray
- Urine MC&S
- CT head (with the justification of an unwitnessed fall, new confusion and on apixaban)

Falls in the elderly are very often multifactorial. See Figure 37.1 for factors to consider.
Initial blood tests show the following (see Table 37.1):

Table 37.1 Venous blood results

Haemoglobin	108 g/L
White cell count	15.7 × 10⁹/L
Neutrophils	10.2 × 10⁹/L
Platelets	391 × 10⁹/L
Sodium	130 mmol/L
Potassium	3.8 mmol/L
Urea	10.8 mmol/L
Creatinine	157 µmol/L
Bilirubin	8 µmol/L
Alanine aminotransferase	27 U/L
Aspartate aminotransferase	26 U/L
Albumin	30 g/L
Glucose	5 mmol/L
CRP	89 mg/L

B12, folate and ferritin are all within normal range.
Chest X-ray shows right-sided lower zone consolidation.
CT head shows no acute findings but some age-related change.

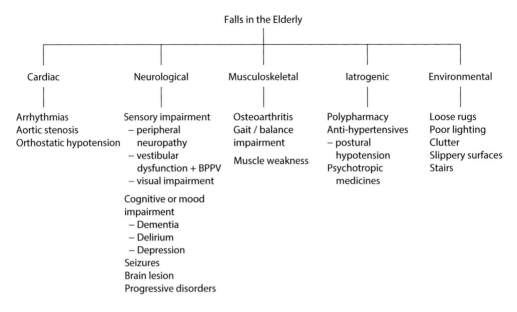

Figure 37.1 Factors to consider in the assessment of falls in the elderly.

Urine culture shows mixed growth, and the CURB-65 score is calculated as 3 (see Further Reading).

What would be the most appropriate management at this stage?

- Start antibiotics for a community-acquired pneumonia
- IV fluids as needed
- Take blood cultures
- Monitor urine output
- Urinary antigens – pneumococcus and legionella
- Oxygen as needed
- Collateral history

Asymptomatic bacteriuria

Asymptomatic bacteriuria is common in the elderly. It does not require treatment and in such patients a urinary tract infection should not be diagnosed based on urine dipstick.

TIMEPOINT ⏱ 2

Three hours after admission, the doctor who had admitted Mrs Atkins sits down with the notes and telephones Mrs Atkins' daughter to obtain a collateral history. Mrs Atkins' daughter reports that she has been increasingly confused over the last week and has reduced mobility compared to normal. Mrs Atkins' daughter describes that she is usually 'very sharp' and has not noted any previous cognitive decline or forgetfulness before the previous week. She usually gets around her bungalow with a frame and still gets out to see friends once a week. Her daughters help her with her shopping, but Mrs Atkins is independent in her activities of daily living.

What is delirium?

Delirium is an acute confusional state. It is common in the elderly, particularly in the presence of infection. The DSM-V diagnostic criteria are as follows:

1. Disturbance in attention (reduced ability to direct, focus, sustain, and shift attention) and awareness

2. The disturbance develops over a short period of time (usually hours to days), represents a change from baseline and tends to fluctuate during the course of the day
3. An additional disturbance in cognition (memory deficit, disorientation, language, visuospatial ability or perception)
4. The disturbances are not better explained by another pre-existing, evolving or established neurocognitive disorder, and do not occur in the context of a severely reduced level of arousal, such as coma
5. There is evidence from the history, physical examination, or laboratory findings that the disturbance is caused by a medical condition, substance intoxication or withdrawal or medication side effect

Delirium can be hyperactive, hypoactive or mixed. Patients with hyperactive delirium may become restless, agitated or aggressive and may demonstrate hallucinations or delusions. In hypoactive delirium, patients tend to be abnormally withdrawn or sleepy which can be easily mistaken for depression. Some people fluctuate between the two with a mixed delirium.

It may take weeks to months for delirium to fully resolve, and is likely to improve further once a patient is back in an environment that is familiar to them, and therefore ongoing confusion should not be a barrier to discharging a patient home provided they will be safe.

A collateral history from relatives or friends who know the patient well can help to establish whether this is a true delirium, or whether there may be a background of slower onset of cognitive decline suggestive of an underlying dementia.

Table 37.2 shows some of the features that relate to delirium compared to dementia.

TIMEPOINT 3

Nine days later, Mrs Atkins is looking much better following antibiotics and is now considered medically stable for discharge. Her delirium has improved significantly. The multidisciplinary team meeting will need to consider a detailed functional assessment and medication review before discharge actually takes place; and in 6–8 weeks post-discharge a 'falls clinic' review is planned.

What other factors may need to be considered before she can be discharged?

- Is she back to her baseline with regards to mobility and activities of daily living?
- Does she need a new package of care to ensure that she is safe and can cope at home?
- What can be done to reduce the risk of falls in the future?

A multidisciplinary team is involved in Mrs Atkins' care including physiotherapy and occupational therapy to assess her mobility, and any help or equipment she may need at home on discharge.

Her current medications are as follows:

Amitriptyline: 10 mg ON
Metformin: 500 mg BD
Bisoprolol: 5 mg OD
Ramipril: 5 mg OD
Furosemide: 40 mg OD
Apixaban: 5 mg BD
Aspirin: 75 mg OD
Levothyroxine: 100 micrograms OD
Laxido: 1 sachet BD
Senna: 7.5 mg OD

Table 37.2 Delirium vs. dementia

Delirium	Dementia
Acute onset over hours to days	Gradual onset over months to years
Fluctuates during the day	Progressive, with little fluctuation
Disturbance in attention and awareness	Attention remains relatively intact
There is evidence of a possible cause	No obvious acute medical cause
Reversible	Irreversible

Mrs Atkins takes a small dose of amitriptyline for back pain. It is decided to gradually reduce this with the aim of stopping it (and replace it with alternative analgesia) to reduce the anticholinergic burden.

What is anticholinergic medication burden?

Anticholinergic drugs are commonly prescribed; however, in older patients they have been correlated with cognitive decline, delirium, physical decline and falls. Single agents with anticholinergic effects may not cause any adverse effects; however, when used in combination, the effect is cumulative. A reduction in anticholingeric burden can help to improve confusion in delirious patients.

Research has shown that each highly anticholinergic drug may increase the risk of cognitive impairment by 46% over 6 years.

Commonly used drugs and their anticholinergic burden are shown in Table 37.3.

Table 37.3 Burden of anticholinergic medications

Highly anticholinergic burden; avoid if possible	Drugs with some anticholinergic activity
Amitriptyline	Atenolol/metoprolol
Chlorphenamine	Cetirizine
Chlorpromazine	Codeine
Clozapine	Colchicine
Olanzapine	Diazepam
Oxybutynin	Digoxin
Quetiapine	Furosemide
Solifenacin	Hydralazine
Tolterodine	Prednisolone
	Ranitidine

TIMEPOINT ⏱ 4

Eight weeks later, at the falls clinic, Mrs Atkins looks much better. Her delirium has completely resolved, and her AMTS is now 10/10. She is managing much better at home; however, she describes a couple of episodes of feeling very dizzy and has had four falls since discharge.

The doctor does a lying/standing blood pressure which reveals a significant postural drop and decides to reduce the dose of bisoprolol and ramipril to reduce the risk of postural hypotension.

What are the major causes of postural hypotension?

- Medication – most commonly antihypertensives, diuretics, nitrates, alpha blockers
- Dehydration
- Anaemia or blood loss
- Addison's disease/adreno-cortical dysfunction
- Autonomic dysfunction – primary such as inherited or acquired autonomic failure; an acquired form in this scenario could be Shy–Drager syndrome; secondary, e.g. diabetes mellitus

The doctor also requests a 72-hour tape (ECG record), which later comes back to show persistent atrial fibrillation, no significant pauses or arrhythmias, and thus a letter is written to Mrs Atkins' address and her GP informing them of that result and suggesting that the current medication remains unchanged.

FURTHER READING

1. http://www.polypharmacy.scot.nhs.uk /polypharmacy-guidance-medicines-re view/for-healthcare-professionals/hot-to pics/anticholinergics/
2. Campbell N, Boustani M, Lane K, et al. Use of anticholinergics and the risk of cognitive impairment in an African-American population. *Neurology*, 2010; 75:152–159.
3. American Psychiatric Association. (2013). *Diagnostic and Statistical Manual of Mental Disorders* (5th ed.). https://doi. org/10.1176/appi.books.9780890425596
4. CURB-65 score: Lim WS, van der Eerden MM, Laing R, et al. Defining community acquired pneumonia severity on presentation to hospital: an international derivation and validation study. *Thorax*, 2003; 58:377–382.

Case 38

Ms Dufe, a 29-year-old woman, comes to see her GP with her 2-month-old son, her second child, for his baby growth check. However, when the GP asks how she is doing, she describes a 10-day history of unexpected breathlessness on minimal exertion such as climbing the stairs or walking 20 metres. There is no history of cough, sputum or haemoptysis. This is concerning to her as she has previously done significant amounts of outdoor sports and finds it very disconcerting to feel breathless on doing minimal activity.

During the first pregnancy, which resulted in her now 3-year-old daughter, she had experienced fatigue, palpitations and breathlessness starting 5 weeks before delivery and ongoing for another 3 months afterwards, although markedly less than currently; she had felt it was 'to be expected' and no investigations were done then.

She has no past medical history and does not take any regular medications. She lives with her husband and 2 children, and works from home for a mental health charity.

Otherwise, from a purely obstetric point of view, both pregnancies themselves had been uncomplicated, the labours were spontaneous and resulted in normal vaginal deliveries. The GP examined her and immediately arranged investigations, via the acute on-call medical team that day.

On arrival at the medical assessment unit, Mrs Dufe is seen by a senior member of the team, who considers a range of possible differential diagnoses. They are aware that a range of cardiac and respiratory disorders, including pulmonary embolism, could cause such a presentation and thus decide to embark upon tests designed to narrow the range of possibilities.

Her observations are as follows:

Respiratory rate: 12/min
Oxygen saturations: 98% on room air
Temperature: 37.1°C
Blood pressure: 127/87 mmHg
Heart rate: 102 bpm

What investigations should be arranged?

- Bloods – FBC, U&E, LFT, D-dimer, CRP, ESR, NT-proBNP
- ECG
- Chest X-ray

All blood tests are normal except for a raised NT-proBNP. The ECG shows sinus tachycardia, and the chest X-ray shows a prominent cardiac outline, with some upper lobe diversion and noticeable vascularity.

What is NT-proBNP?

NT-proBNP is the inactive fragment of a hormone released by the heart when the ventricles are stretched, for example by fluid overload. The hormone causes fluid and sodium loss in the urine and mild vasodilation. Thus, in theory, a natriuretic peptide would generate natriuresis, utilising a renal mechanism that would ensure salt and fluid loss as a physiological response to the sensation of fluid overload. The serum levels of NT-proBNP have been validated in laboratory assays for diagnostic purposes. NT-proBNP levels are raised in heart failure and increase in level according to the New York Heart Association classification. If NT-proBNP is normal, it has a potential to help reduce the chance of there being heart failure present – with an approximate negative predictive value of 97%.

When should a request for an NT-proBNP test be made?

The NICE guidance recommends that NT-proBNP is measured in patients with suspected heart failure. Very high levels of NT-proBNP are associated with a poor prognosis. Refer patients with NT-proBNP >2000 ng/L for urgent assessment and echocardiography within 2 weeks. Refer patients with NT-proBNP between 400–2000 ng/L for assessment and echocardiography within 6 weeks. NTproBNP levels <400 ng/litre mean heart failure is unlikely. Levels do not help to distinguish heart failure with or without a preserved ejection fraction.

Is there anything else that can affect NT-proBNP levels?

See Table 38.1.

TIMEPOINT ⏱ 2

Mrs Dufe is set up to attend a hot clinic cardiology outpatients the next day. This is a newly developed one-stop service that integrates obstetric physicians, cardiac specialist nurses, cardiologists and cardiac technicians.

On arrival, Mrs Dufe's observations are:

Respiratory rate: 16/min
Oxygen saturations: 95% on room air
Temperature: 37.0°C
Blood pressure: 133/76 mmHg
Heart rate: 93 bpm

Mrs Dufe is assessed clinically and an echocardiogram takes place in the cardiac centre, prior to the final clinical consultation.

The echocardiogram shows reduced ejection fraction of 34% but no obvious hypertrophic changes to the myocardial/septal areas, nothing more than trivial regurgitation and no significant stenotic valvular findings.

Table 38.1 Factors affecting NT-proBNP levels

Increase NT-proBNP	Decrease NT-proBNP
Left ventricular hypertrophy	Obesity
Right ventricular overload	Diuretics
Ischaemia	ACE inhibitors
Hypoxaemia	Beta-blockers
PE	Angiotensin receptor antagonists
Sepsis	Aldosterone antagonists
COPD	
Diabetes	
Liver cirrhosis	
Age >70	
eGFR <60 mL/min	

The attending cardiologist concludes that Mrs Dufe has peripartum cardiomyopathy (PPCM) and informs her as to the best steps for monitoring and managing her condition.

What is peripartum cardiomyopathy (PPCM), and how is it treated?

Peripartum cardiomyopathy is a condition of cardiac dysfunction taking place in the period around delivery and for several months afterwards. Key features are as follows:

- Reduced cardiac output
- Increased filling pressures
- The ejection fraction is nearly always reduced below 45%
- In future pregnancies, cardiac dysfunction may recur in the peri- and postpartum state
- Risk factors
  - Pre-eclampsia
  - Twin pregnancy
  - Afro-Caribbean ethnicity

Subsequent pregnancies can be linked with a worse outcome, especially when left ventricular structure and function did not completely recover in the first episode.

Treatment of this condition is predominantly similar to other medical therapy for cardiac dysfunction, but more disease-modifying treatments are hoped to be developed. One theory is that prolactin is a key factor in this disease, and therefore the attempt to use bromocriptine (a prolactin inhibitor) is one option being considered. The list of future or potential treatments for this condition is therefore as follows:

- Prolactin inhibitor, e.g. bromocriptine
- Anti-VEGF drugs
- Perhexiline
- Pentoxifylline
- Serelaxin
- Antisense oligonucleotides

Mrs Dufe is asked if she is breast or bottle feeding. In the absence of breast feeding, and on appropriate contraception (see below), medication is initiated to provide symptomatic relief, as per for any cause of left ventricular dysfunction.

Contraception options in PPCM

Coil devices (either copper only or with progestogen), progesterone implants, injectable progesterone or progesterone-only pills are the preferred types of contraception. Oral contraceptives containing oestrogen are not recommended, because they are prothrombotic and barrier methods are not regarded as sufficiently reliable.

The specialist nurse spends time after the clinic reassuring and supporting Mrs Dufe as to the means to monitor and treat her condition and invites her to participate in the development of an information leaflet on the condition.

TIMEPOINT ⏱ 3

Three months later, Mrs Dufe attends the scheduled cardiology outpatients. She feels much better. The echocardiogram done on this clinic visit still shows a slightly reduced (but much improved) ejection fraction of 46% with no other new findings. The consultation on this occasion focuses on titrating the diuretic and other medication downwards given her improving condition and setting up virtual clinic plans for ongoing follow-up to continue the process of modifying the treatment as needed over time.

It is clear that at this stage, Mrs Dufe does not need any further 'next-step' interventional treatment strategies, but when asked by one of the medical students in clinic, the cardiologist lists the potential technologies that could be used if a cardiomyopathy, for reasons of rhythm alteration or cardiac function variation, necessitated doing so.

What are the non-medical management options for cardiomyopathies?

- Wearable cardioverter defibrillators
- Implantable cardioverter defibrillators
- Left ventricular assist devices
- Cardiac transplantation

TIMEPOINT ⏱ 4

Three years later, Mrs Dufe attends a further cardiology outpatient appointment. She has 'open access' to the clinic based on pre-specified criteria, one of which is for people with a previous episode of PPCM – returning to the clinic is welcomed in those who are pregnant or considering further pregnancies. Mrs Dufe is now 7 weeks pregnant again, but she is fearful the symptoms will recur, given that the situation has happened twice before. Thus, she is immediately referred into the obstetric/medical/cardiac combined clinic service, which she will remain associated with throughout the antenatal and postnatal periods.

How likely is it that she has made a complete recovery from her previous episode of PPCM?

PPCM is one of the cardiomyopathy conditions with the highest likelihood of complete or near-complete recovery.

FURTHER READING

1. https://heart.bmj.com/content/early/2017/11/09/heartjnl-2016-310599?hwoasp=authn%3A1535398525%3A5531150%3A1543610769%3A0%3A0%3A2vlmRtggzzeQWvb9XAyBlA%3D%3D

2. https://www.bmj.com/content/bmj/364/bmj.k5287.full.pdf

3. http://www.clinmed.rcpjournal.org/content/17/4/316.full

4. https://www.nice.org.uk/guidance/ng106

Case 39

TIMEPOINT 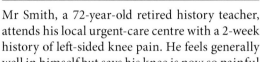 1

Mr Smith, a 72-year-old retired history teacher, attends his local urgent-care centre with a 2-week history of left-sided knee pain. He feels generally well in himself but says his knee is now so painful he can barely walk, when usually he is very active and enjoys going for long walks in the country-side with his wife.

He has also noticed that his left knee has started to appear a little red and swollen over the last few days. The right knee is completely nor-mal, and he does not have pain in any of his other joints. He denies having any fevers and confirms that he has never had anything like this before.

His past medical history includes atrial fibril-lation, hypertension and a cholecystectomy aged 45. He takes bisoprolol, warfarin and ramipril and has no known drug allergies. He lives at home with his wife. He usually mobilises inde-pendently and can do all his activities of daily liv-ing. He does not smoke or drink alcohol.

On examination, his observations are normal.

His left knee is warm and erythematous compared to the right side. It is tender to pal-pation. There is an obvious effusion with a positive patellar tap. His range of movement is limited to ≈20 degrees both actively and pas-sively. Neurovascular examination is normal. He is clearly modifying his gait in order to avoid weight-bearing through the left knee.

The urgent-care doctor requests blood tests and an X-ray of the left knee.

His point of care INR is 2.3, so the doctor proceeds with aspiration of the knee effusion (arthrocentesis). The fluid appears cloudy and yellow. It is sent to the lab for analysis.

Which blood tests should be sent and why?

- Full blood count – to look for raised white cells indicative of infection or inflammation
- Urea and electrolytes – useful as a baseline to assess renal function before starting any new medications
- Liver function tests – useful as a baseline to assess liver function before starting any new medications
- Coagulation screen – the patient is on warfa-rin, so it would be reasonable to monitor his INR at this contact with a medical profes-sional, in order to adjust his warfarin dosing if needed
- CRP and ESR – if raised, may be suggestive of an infectious or inflammatory process
- Urate – high urate levels may suggest a diag-nosis of gout
- Rheumatoid factor and anti-CCP – to screen for a possible new diagnosis of rheumatoid arthritis

What are the key features distinguishing osteoarthritis, gout and pseudogout on X-ray?

See Table 39.1.

The X-ray demonstrates some subchondral cysts, but otherwise appears normal.

The urgent-care doctor discharges Mr Smith with analgesia and promises to phone with the results of the aspiration, advising that they should be available within the week.

Table 39.1 Factors distinguishing osteoarthritis, gout and pseudogout on X-ray

	Osteoarthritis	Gout	Pseudogout
Joint space loss	✓	Preserved until late stage	
Osteophytes	✓		
Subchondral cysts	✓		✓
Subchondral sclerosis	✓		
Erosions	✓	✓ ('Rat bite' erosions – overhanging sclerotic margins)	
Lytic lesions		✓	
Effusions		✓	
Chondrocalcinosis			✓

What are the features of aspiration for the differential diagnoses?

See Table 39.2.

Management of gout and pseudogout

Gout	Pseudogout

• First line = NSAIDs
• Second line = colchicine
• Third line = oral steroids
• PLUS analgesia
• Prophylaxis = allopurinol, febuxostat, sulfinpyrazone
	• Any symptomatic treatment, e.g.
	  • Ice
	  • NSAIDs
	  • Joint aspiration
	  • Intra-articular steroid injection
	  • Oral steroids

TIMEPOINT ⏰ 2

Three days later, Mr Smith, feeling very unwell, presents to the emergency department accompanied by his wife. He says that his knee pain is even worse than before, and he feels 'terrible'. He denies having any chest or urinary symptoms.

On examination he looks sweaty and unwell.

His observations are:

Respiratory rate: 28/min
Oxygen saturations: 97% on room air
Temperature: 39.4°C
Blood pressure: 135/92 mmHg
Heart rate: 102 bpm

On examination, his left knee appears erythematous and extremely swollen. It is warm to touch. His wife reports that both the redness and swelling are significantly worse than earlier in the week, and Mr Smith agrees.

His systems examination is within normal limits.

Results from 3 days prior show:

Venous blood results

White cell count	14.0×10^9/L
CRP	89 mg/L
Urate	323 µmol/L

Knee joint aspiration: positively birefringent rhombus shaped crystals, suggestive of pseudogout

Urate levels

Urate levels may be normal in an acute attack of gout.

Table 39.2 Interpretation of joint aspiration results

	Colour	Appearance	White cell count	Urate	Polarised light	Culture	Glucose
Normal	Colourless-pale yellow	Transparent	<200 cells/mm^3	Neg	Neg	Neg	= serum
Septic	Yellow-green	Cloudy/opaque	>50,000 cells/mm^3	Neg	Neg	Pos	Less than serum
Gout	Yellow	Cloudy	2000–50,000 cells/mm^3	Pos	Needle-shaped crystals, blue. Negative birefringence	Neg	Less than serum
Pseudogout	Yellow	Cloudy	2000–50,000 cells/mm^3	Neg	Rhombus-shaped crystals, yellow. Positive birefringence	Neg	Less than serum

The doctor repeats his blood tests and sends blood cultures.

Mr Smith's results today demonstrate:

Venous blood results

White cell count	19.2×10^9/L
CRP	230 mg/L

The doctor explains to Mr Smith that he thinks he is suffering from a septic arthritis, secondary to the aspiration of his knee done in the urgent-care centre.

What risks should you counsel the patient on when consenting to joint aspiration?

- Pain
- Infection
- Bleeding, bruising and haemarthrosis
- Damage to local structures, such as nerves and vessels
- Allergic reactions or side effects from any injected steroid
- Failure of procedure

Key point

Anticoagulation with warfarin is NOT a contraindication for joint aspiration.

The doctor repeats Mr Smith's joint aspiration and sends it for Gram staining and repeat cultures.

He then starts Mr Smith on IV flucloxacillin 2 g QDS, as per local trust guidelines.

TIMEPOINT ⏱ 3

Mr Smith remains in the majors section of the emergency department, awaiting a bed on the wards.

Seven hours later, the emergency buzzer goes off for his bed.

The nurse is still standing there as he has just given Mr Smith his second dose of IV flucloxacillin. He is not known to have any drug allergies.

Mr Smith appears pale, is very short of breath and appears to be in respiratory distress. He has obvious swelling around his lips.

His observations are:

Respiratory rate: 44/min
Oxygen saturations: 86% on room air
Temperature: 38.6°C
Blood pressure: 73/49 mmHg
Heart rate: 93 bpm

What is the likeliest diagnosis?

Anaphylaxis to penicillin.

How should this be managed immediately?

- 2222/peri-arrest call – urgent anaesthetic input is required to manage airway swelling
- STOP the drug
- Give 15 L/min of high-flow oxygen via a non-rebreathe mask
- Adrenaline IM, 500 micrograms of 1:1000
- 0.9% sodium chloride IV, 1 litre STAT fluid challenge
- Chlorphenamine IM or slow IV, 10 mg
- Hydrocortisone IM or slow IV, 200 mg
- Reassess DRABCDE in full

What precautions should be taken to avoid this happening again?

- Clearly state penicillin anaphylaxis on patient's drug chart
- Give Mr Smith a wristband to identify his penicillin allergy
- Update alerts on any electronic systems to identify Mr Smith's penicillin allergy
- Include information regarding the allergy in Mr Smith's discharge letter
- Change the antibiotic to an appropriate alternative according to your local trust guidelines. Discuss with the microbiology team if necessary

Table 39.3 Cytochrome P450 inducers and inhibitors

Cytochrome P450 inducers	Cytochrome P450 inhibitors
REDUCE concentration of warfarin	INCREASE concentration of warfarin
Anticoagulant effect of warfarin REDUCED	Anticoagulant effect of warfarin INCREASES
INR DECREASES	INR INCREASES
INCREASED risk of thromboembolism	INCREASED risk of bleeding
e.g.	e.g.
• Carbamazepine • Griseofulvin • Phenobarbital • Phenytoin • Rifampicin • St John's Wort	• Amiodarone • Chloramphenicol • Cimetidine • Ciprofloxacin • Clarithromycin • Erythromycin • Fluconazole • Fluoxetine • Grapefruit juice • Isoniazid • Ketoconazole • Metronidazole • Omeprazole • Sodium valproate • Sulphonamides

Mr Smith is started on ciprofloxacin as per the advice of the consultant microbiologist.

Mr Smith recovers well from the episode of anaphylaxis. He remains in hospital for a further week to receive IV ciprofloxacin, and then is discharged with another 5 weeks of tablets to take at home.

TIMEPOINT ⏱ 4

Eight days later, Mr Smith returns to the emergency department again as he has a nosebleed from his left nostril which has lasted for over 3 hours, despite him attempting to squeeze firmly on the bottom part of his nose.

He is haemodynamically stable.

The doctor in the emergency department applies an ice pack for 20 minutes but this does not stem the bleeding. She therefore refers to ENT who attend and cauterise his left nostril with silver nitrate.

The emergency department doctor also sends off routine bloods.

What is the sequence of events that has led to Mr Smith having a nosebleed of this severity?

- Mr Smith was started on ciprofloxacin for the treatment of his septic arthritis once his anaphylaxis to penicillin was discovered
- Ciprofloxacin is a cytochrome P450 inhibitor (Table 39.3)
- This means that it increases the anticoagulant effect of warfarin, increasing Mr Smith's INR so that it is supratherapeutic and predisposing Mr Smith to excessive bleeding

Mr Smith's results today show:

Venous blood results

White cell count	15.4×10^9/L
CRP	184 mg/L
INR	6.8

Table 39.4 Management of raised INR

Situation	Vitamin K dose	Warfarin
INR 5–8 + minor bleeding	1–3 mg slow IV	Stop warfarin + restart when INR <5
INR >8 + no bleeding	1–5 mg PO Repeat dose if INR still too high after 24 hours	
INR >8 + minor bleeding	1–3 mg slow IV Repeat dose if INR still too high after 24 hours	
Major bleed in warfarinised patient	5 mg IV	Stop warfarin

How should a patient with a high INR be managed?

See Table 39.4.

As Mr Smith's INR is 6.8, the doctor crosses off his warfarin, gives him 3 mg of vitamin K IV and includes a plan in the notes that the warfarin should be restarted when his INR is less than 5 again (titrated cautiously). He continues the course of ciprofloxacin as there is no better alternative for the treatment of his septic joint. The doctor also suggests that Mr Smith consider whether it would be worth changing from warfarin to a different type of anticoagulation, such as a DOAC, which might be easier for him to use. The doctor provides Mr Smith with an information leaflet which he agrees to read.

Case 40

Ms West is a 36-year-old solicitor who attends her GP as she has been finding it increasingly difficult to type over the last 8 weeks, due to pain and stiffness in her fingers. It has now reached the point where it is slowing her down at work. She is concerned that if she doesn't meet her upcoming deadlines, she will not be considered for a promotion, which is why she has come for advice. The GP asks if there are any other symptoms that she is concerned about. Ms West explains that she has been quite stiff lately, and as a result has been getting up half an hour earlier in the morning to make it easier to do her make-up. Ms West also mentions that she has struggled to open jars recently as this is quite painful, and she has generally felt a bit unwell, almost as if she has flu. She also thinks that her fingers might be a bit puffy, but can't decide if she is imagining this.

Ms West has a background of bipolar disease which has been stable for many years on lithium (Priadel) 1 g OD. She has no known drug allergies. She smokes around ten cigarettes a day but rarely drinks alcohol as she hates being hungover. She lives with her long-term boyfriend and their 3-year-old daughter.

Her observations are:

Respiratory rate: 16/min
Oxygen saturations: 98% on room air
Temperature: 36.3°C
Blood pressure: 113/76 mmHg
Heart rate: 65 bpm

On examination of the hands, she has evidence of symmetrical, active synovitis in eight out of ten metacarpophalangeal joints, and six out of ten proximal interphalangeal joints. Nine of the small joints of the hands are tender. She also has a positive metacarpophalangeal joint squeeze test. A fine tremor is noted. Her systems examination is otherwise unremarkable.

The GP is concerned about a possible new onset inflammatory arthritis.

Which tests should the GP request and why?

- Full blood count: raised white cells, baseline required if starting DMARDs
- Urea and electrolytes: baseline required if starting DMARDs
- Liver function tests: baseline required if starting DMARDs
- C-reactive protein: evidence of inflammation
- Erythrocyte sedimentation rate (ESR): evidence of inflammation
- Rheumatoid factor: supports diagnosis of rheumatoid arthritis if positive
- Anti-cyclic citrullinated peptide (anti-CCP) autoantibodies: supports diagnosis of rheumatoid arthritis if positive
- Plain X-rays of the hands and feet: to look for evidence of erosions or other joint damage

The GP explains his concerns to Ms West and advises her to take regular paracetamol and ibuprofen to help manage her pain until the results are back from her initial tests. Ms West asks if she needs to see a specialist or not. The GP thinks that it probably isn't necessary but agrees to double-check the current referral criteria.

Should this referral be classed as urgent?

Yes, as Ms West has a persistent synovitis affecting the small joints of her hands.

The current NICE guidelines recommend that any adult with suspected persistent synovitis should be referred urgently for a specialist opinion if:

- The small joints of the hands or feet are affected
- More than one joint is affected
- It has been more than 3 months since symptoms began

This advice applies even if they have normal CRP, ESR, rheumatoid factor or anti-CCP tests.

The GP agrees that Ms West does fit the criteria and promises to do an urgent rheumatology referral later that evening.

Seronegative rheumatoid arthritis

Rheumatoid arthritis may still be diagnosed even in the absence of positive rheumatoid factor or anti-CCP antibodies. This is known as seronegative disease, and includes around 30% of the rheumatoid arthritis cohort. Antibodies sometimes develop many years after the initial diagnosis so the patient becomes seropositive.

Seropositive patients are thought to have slightly more severe disease, and may also respond better to certain treatments. However, the overall evidence suggests that antibody titres do not necessarily correlate well with disease activity.

TIMEPOINT ⏱ 2

One week later, Ms West is brought to the emergency department by her boyfriend. Over the last 48 hours she has had worsening diarrhoea and vomiting. She still has a lot of pain in her hands, so she has continued to take paracetamol 1 g QDS and ibuprofen 400 mg TDS all week. However, her boyfriend is more concerned about the fact that she doesn't seem to be able to walk in a straight line, and she seems very shaky. Ms West keeps repeating that she needs to go to visit her mother

and check that she is ok, but Ms West's boyfriend says that her mother passed away many years ago. Ms West nearly falls as she transfers between the wheelchair and the examination couch, saying that 'everything seems blurry'.

Her observations are:

Respiratory rate: 22/min
Oxygen saturations: 97% on room air
Temperature: 37.7°C
Blood pressure: 98/73 mmHg
Heart rate: 97 bpm

On examination, Ms West is clearly confused and is not orientated to time, place or person. Her cardiovascular, respiratory and abdominal examinations are all unremarkable. Cranial nerve examination is normal except for reduced visual acuity due to the visual blurring. Eye movements, visual fields and fundoscopy are all normal.

On neurological examination of the limbs, tone is normal and power is 4 out of 5 in all regions examined. There are brisk reflexes throughout and a coarse resting tremor is observed. Ms West's coordination is distinctly poor, and her gait is ataxic when she is asked to mobilise.

The emergency department doctor is unsure as to what might be causing this picture. He sends some routine blood tests, including a confusion screen, and requests a chest X-ray and urine dip to look for any obvious signs of infection. He asks the nurses to continue to observe Ms West until the test results come back and goes to discuss the case with his consultant.

What is the most likely diagnosis and what has led to this happening?

Ms West has developed lithium toxicity secondary to taking regular ibuprofen over the last week. Ibuprofen interacts with lithium leading to accumulation and toxicity.

Important symptoms include:

- Vomiting and diarrhoea
- Visual disturbance
- Confusion and drowsiness
- Neurological abnormalities, e.g. weakness, myoclonus, poor coordination, ataxia, abnormal reflexes

- Incontinence
- Coarse tremor

Tremor in patients taking lithium

- **Fine tremor** = the patient is fine – side effect of lithium at therapeutic doses
- **Coarse tremor** = cause for concern – sign of lithium toxicity

---

Severe toxicity may result in arrhythmias, seizures, renal failure, coma and death.

The consultant reviews Ms West's history and points out that the ibuprofen might have interacted with her lithium. He asks the emergency department doctor to request that a lithium level be added on to the bloods that have already been sent, and to start IV fluids and commence cardiac monitoring while he is waiting for the results.

Blood results are shown in Table 40.1.

How should Ms West be managed immediately?

- Hold the lithium
- A full panel of blood tests including a full blood count, urea and electrolytes, liver function tests, calcium levels and thyroid function tests
- Lithium levels should be checked immediately on admission and then 6-hourly until stable
- An ECG should be performed to look for abnormal QRS complexes, a prolonged QT interval or arrhythmias and cardiac monitoring commenced if possible

- The mainstay of treatment is IV fluids to treat dehydration, electrolyte imbalances and kidney injury
- Any other symptoms such as seizures or arrhythmias should be managed as per usual protocols
- Severe cases may require gastric lavage, whole bowel irrigation or haemodialysis
- Activated charcoal should **not** be used as it does not adsorb lithium and diuretics should not be given
- Advice should be sought from senior staff as the patient may need to be transferred to higher level care
- In any case of poisoning or overdose, consult Toxbase.org or phone the UK National Poisons Information Service helpline

The emergency department doctor requests an ECG and prescribes another bag of IV fluids given the acute kidney injury and hypernatraemia.

Ms West's chest X-ray, urine dip and ECG are all normal.

The emergency department doctor notices that Ms West's lithium level is 1.8 mmol/L, confirming moderate toxicity.

He phones the UK National Poisons Information Service helpline who advise that haemodialysis should be considered given the presence of neurological symptoms. The emergency department doctor consults with the renal registrar who accepts Ms West for emergency haemodialysis via a central line. Ms West's symptoms improve over the next 48 hours, and her blood tests are repeated at this point (Table 40.2).

When Ms West is seen again on the ward round, she asks when her lithium can be restarted as she is worried about her bipolar symptoms coming back.

Table 40.1 Venous blood results

White cell count	8.3 × 10⁹/L	Corrected calcium	2.42 mmol/L
Haemoglobin	107 g/L	Magnesium	0.82 mmol/L
Platelets	293 × 10⁹/L	CRP	17 mg/L
MCV	85 fL	Albumin	42 g/L
Sodium	152 mmol/L	Bilirubin	10 μmol/L
Potassium	4.4 mmol/L	Alkaline phosphatase	48 U/L
Urea	7.5 mmol/L	Alanine aminotransferase	23 U/L
Creatinine	157 μmol/L		

Table 40.2 Venous blood results

White cell count	4.7×10^9/L	Corrected calcium	2.22 mmol/L
Haemoglobin	106 g/L	Magnesium	0.88 mmol/L
Platelets	303×10^9/L	CRP	22 mg/L
MCV	86 fL	Albumin	43 g/L
Sodium	144 mmol/L	Bilirubin	12 µmol/L
Potassium	4.2 mmol/L	Alkaline phosphatase	46 U/L
Urea	5.3 mmol/L	Alanine aminotransferase	28 U/L
Creatinine	83 µmol/L	Lithium	0.92 mmol/L

When should lithium be restarted after an episode of toxicity?

Lithium levels need to be monitored (ideally 6-hourly) until levels are stable and any symptoms of diarrhoea and vomiting have settled. Lithium can be restarted once it is back within the therapeutic range (0.4–1 mmol/L).

Lithium interactions

Lithium interacts with many over-the-counter and commonly prescribed medications, including:

- NSAIDs
- ACE-inhibitors
- Angiotensin-II receptor antagonists
- Thiazide diuretics
- SSRIs

Toxicity may also be provoked easily by dehydration due to the drug's narrow therapeutic range.

The renal doctors explain that as her lithium levels are now within the therapeutic range again, she can restart her lithium tablets. They give her a leaflet explaining more about lithium toxicity and which medications can precipitate this to avoid her having the same problem in the future. She is discharged home later that day.

TIMEPOINT ⏱ 3

Two days later, Ms West is seen in the rheumatology clinic.

The initial blood tests sent by the GP are checked by the rheumatologist (Table 40.3).

The rheumatologist examines Ms West and agrees with the GP's assessment that she has 14 swollen and 9 tender joints in the hands. He assesses the rest of her joints and is satisfied that they are unaffected. He reviews her X-rays which demonstrate some soft tissue swelling but no bony abnormalities. The rheumatologist asks Ms West to rate her 'global health score', with 0 being the best and 100 being the worst. Ms West rates her current health as 80 on the scale.

Table 40.3 Venous blood results

White cell count	5.9×10^9/L	ESR	54 mm/hr
Haemoglobin	105 g/L	CRP	18 mg/L
Platelets	352×10^9/L	Albumin	43 g/L
MCV	86 fL	Bilirubin	12 µmol/L
Sodium	143 mmol/L	Alkaline phosphatase	46 U/L
Potassium	5.1 mmol/L	Alanine aminotransferase	28 U/L
Urea	4.8 mmol/L	Rheumatoid factor	493 IU/mL
Creatinine	78 µmol/L	Anti-CCP	195 U/mL

The rheumatologist calculates that her DAS28 score is 6.64, suggestive of high disease activity.

DAS28 scoring in rheumatoid arthritis

The DAS28 is a disease activity score used to monitor disease severity and response to treatment in rheumatoid arthritis. It is a validated score that is calculated using the following components:

- Tender and swollen joints out of 28 joints assessed (shoulders, elbows, wrists, knees, all MCP joints and PIP joints)
- ESR
- Patient global health rating on a scale from 0 (best) to 100 (worst)

Depending on how much the DAS28 score improves between two timepoints, it can be demonstrated that the disease has shown a good response, moderate response or no response to the treatment trialled.

The rheumatologist advises that Ms West should start on 7.5 mg of oral methotrexate weekly. He arranges for her to have a phone call with the rheumatology specialist nurse the following week to see how things are going, and then blood tests and a follow-up appointment in 2 weeks.

What monitoring is required for methotrexate?

- Each blood test should include a full blood count, urea and electrolytes including an eGFR, and liver function tests including ALT and albumin
- Bloods need to be checked
  - Until the patient has been on a stable dose for 6 weeks
    - Every 2 weeks
  - Once the patient is on a stable dose
    - Once a month for 3 months

- Once every 3 months thereafter

What additional considerations are there for a patient newly prescribed methotrexate, aside from blood monitoring?

Patients should receive clear explanations of the following:

- Methotrexate is a medication that is given **once weekly**, and should always be taken on the same day each week to avoid confusion
- Folic acid will need to be co-prescribed (5 mg once weekly, to be taken on a different day to the methotrexate), which helps to reduce some of the methotrexate side effects
- Patients must ensure that they attend for their blood monitoring, and should use the purple methotrexate monitoring book to document their weekly dose and blood results
- Patients should be aware not to use aspirin, ibuprofen or other NSAIDs when using methotrexate, as taking both increases the risk of nephrotoxicity and methotrexate toxicity
- Patients should be aware of possible symptoms that may be a feature of severe disease secondary to methotrexate, for example
  - Sore throat, bruising and mouth ulcers may be features of bone marrow suppression
  - Nausea, vomiting, abdominal pain and dark urine may be features of liver toxicity
- Patients should be aware that they will require pneumococcus and annual influenza vaccinations
- Patients should be aware that the methotrexate may need to be held if they become unwell with a serious infection

TIMEPOINT 🕐 4

Four months later, Ms West sees her GP as she is concerned that she may be pregnant. She vaguely remembered being told that she should tell her

GP if she became pregnant whilst taking both the lithium and the methotrexate. She had awakened feeling nauseous every morning of the previous week and hadn't been using any contraception so thought she should take a pregnancy test to check. She took two pregnancy tests at home and had one positive and one negative result, so she didn't know what to do.

The nurse checks a urine pregnancy test, which is negative, but advises that as she has had a positive pregnancy test today it would be safest to check a serum βHCG to be completely sure.

What are the considerations when prescribing methotrexate to women of childbearing age?

- Methotrexate is teratogenic and should not be given in pregnancy
- Effective contraception is required during treatment **and** for at least 3 months after treatment has been stopped
- This advice currently applies to men as well, as there is not enough evidence at present that it is definitely safe for male partners who wish to conceive
- Fertility may be reduced during therapy, but this effect is thought to be reversible
- Women who accidentally become pregnant whilst taking methotrexate should be offered extra support from a fetal medicine specialist
- High-dose folate (5 mg daily) should be used instead of the standard dose (400 micrograms daily) for neural tube defect prophylaxis
- Methotrexate is present in breast milk so women should not breastfeed whilst using it

What are the considerations when prescribing lithium to women of childbearing age?

- Lithium should be avoided in women hoping to become pregnant if there is any other option that is suitable to manage their mental health
- Lithium is teratogenic if used in the first trimester. There is a high risk of cardiac defects, especially Ebstein's anomaly

- Women of childbearing age taking lithium should be aware of the need to use effective contraception
- If a woman already taking lithium becomes pregnant
  - If she is well and not at high risk of relapse
    - Consider stopping the drug gradually over 4 weeks
    - Be aware that this is unlikely to significantly alter the risk of cardiac malformations and carries a risk of relapse
  - If she is not well, or at high risk of relapse, consider
    - Switching gradually to an antipsychotic OR
    - Stopping lithium and restarting it in the second trimester OR
    - Continuing the lithium if the woman is at high risk of relapse and no other medication is likely to be effective
- If the woman remains on lithium during the pregnancy, be aware that
  - Her dose requirement may be increased during the second and third trimesters
  - She will require careful monitoring of her lithium levels throughout
- Once the baby is born
  - Be aware of the risk of toxicity in the neonate
  - Women should avoid breastfeeding as lithium is present in the milk

The GP confirms that the serum βHCG is negative, so Ms West is definitely not pregnant. Ms West is very relieved. She asks about the other forms of contraception that are available to her as she has only ever used barrier methods before, and she is now very worried about accidentally becoming pregnant whilst using methotrexate and lithium. She would like to know what the GP would recommend for her.

Which options for contraception should Ms West be counselled about? What are the key points that the GP should make Ms West aware of?

- Factors that need to be considered include the patient's age, smoking status, medical history, any medications they use, personal preference and likelihood of compliance with a daily pill
- The UK Medical Eligibility Criteria for Contraceptive Use (UKMEC), published by the Faculty of Sexual and Reproductive Healthcare, gives information on whether each type of contraception is safe according to the patient's personal characteristics and past medical history. It does not advise on the best or most effective method. Efficacy data are available separately, and the best method must take into account the patient's preference
- A UKMEC category is assigned to each characteristic and condition
  - UKMEC 1: no restriction
  - UKMEC 2: advantages generally outweigh the theoretical or proven risks
  - UKMEC 3: theoretical or proven risks usually outweigh the advantages. Not usually recommended unless other more appropriate methods are not available or acceptable
  - UKMEC 4: represents an unacceptable health risk
- The basic options available to any patient are
  - Intrauterine contraceptives (long-acting reversible contraception)
    - Copper-containing intrauterine contraceptive device (copper coil)
    - Levonorgestrel releasing intrauterine system (e.g. Mirena® or Jaydess®)
  - Progestogen-only contraception
    - Implant
    - Depot injection
    - Progestogen-only pill
  - Combined hormonal contraception
    - Combined oral pill
    - Transdermal patches
    - Vaginal rings

- Patients must be aware that none of these methods offer protection against sexually transmitted infections, including HIV
- The following considerations may be relevant for Ms West (a 36-year-old current smoker [10 cigarettes/day] with rheumatoid arthritis and bipolar disease)
  - The intrauterine contraceptives may be a good option for longer-term contraception if Ms West feels that her family is complete, or if she is not planning to have more children soon. This is particularly relevant for a patient taking two medications which are known teratogens
  - Non-oral contraceptives may be a better option in a patient who may have poor compliance, or may forget to use a daily pill
  - Age 36: UKMEC1 for all forms of contraception
  - Smoker 10/day
    - Intrauterine contraceptives = UKMEC 1 irrespective of smoking status
    - Progestogen-only contraceptives = UKMEC 1 irrespective of smoking status
    - Combined hormonal contraceptives (due to risk of cardiovascular disease and myocardial infarction) =
      - Current smoker, age <35 years = UKMEC 2
      - Current smoker, age ≥35 years =
        - <15 cigarettes/day = UKMEC 3
        - ≥15 cigarettes/day = UKMEC 4
  - Rheumatoid arthritis
    - Copper coil = UKMEC 1
    - All other forms of contraception UKMEC 2 due to increased cardiovascular risk
  - Bipolar disease: no data available for any form of contraception
- Therefore, given Ms West's age, smoking status, rheumatoid arthritis and current use of teratogenic medications, the safest and most appropriate contraceptive option for her would probably be the copper coil

- Ms West would need to be counselled on the risks of using a copper coil including expulsion, infection, uterine perforation and increased risk of ectopic pregnancy. She should also be aware of the side effects including menorrhagia and dysmenorrhoea (especially as she is unable to use ibuprofen as it interacts with lithium and methotrexate). If these side effects are unacceptable to her, then other options should be explained and discussed

Ms West thanks the GP for her time and says that she is happy to go ahead with the copper coil. She does not want to risk accidentally becoming pregnant on methotrexate and lithium and is happy that she has completed her family, so agrees that one of the intrauterine contraceptives would be a good idea. She wants to avoid all the hormonal contraceptives due to the increased cardiovascular risk. As she has always had very light periods in the past, Ms West is sure that she would be able to manage even if the coil does make her periods a little heavier and more painful. The GP blocks out a longer appointment for the following week so that Ms West can come back to have a copper coil inserted. The GP gives Ms West an information leaflet and reassures her that she can change her mind at any time, and to be in touch if she has any further questions.

FURTHER READING

1. FSRH UK Medical Eligibility Criteria for Contraceptive Use (UK MEC). https://www.fsrh.org/ukmec/

List of Abbreviations

βHCG	Beta human chorionic gonadotropin
A&E	Accident and Emergency Department
ABG	Arterial blood gas
ACE	Angiotensin-converting enzyme
ACS	Acute coronary syndrome
ADPKD	Adult polycystic kidney disease
AF	Atrial fibrillation
AFP	Alpha fetoprotein
AIDS	Acquired immunodeficiency syndrome
AKI	Acute kidney injury
ALP	Alkaline phosphatase
ALS	Advanced life support
ALT	Alanine aminotransferase
AMTS	Abbreviated Mental Test Score
ANA	Antinuclear antibodies
ANCA	Antineutrophil cytoplasmic antibodies
AP	Anteroposterior
APTT	Activated partial thromboplastin time
APTTR	Activated partial thromboplastin time ratio
ASD	Atrial septal defect
AST	Aspartate transaminase
AV	Aortic valve
AVPU	Alert, Verbal, Pain, Unresponsive – level of consciousness scale
b.d., bd, BD	Twice a day

BLS	Basic life support
BMI	Body mass index
BNO	Bowels not open
BNP	Brain natriuretic peptide
BO	Bowels open
BP	Blood pressure
BPPV	Benign paroxysmal positional vertigo
BRCA	BReast CAncer gene
CABG	Coronary artery bypass graft
CAD	Coronary artery disease
CCP	Cyclic citrullinated peptide
CD	Crohn's disease
CEA	Carcinoembryonic antigen
CK	Creatine kinase
CKD	Chronic kidney disease
CMHN	Community mental health nurse
CMV	Cytomegalovirus
CNS	Central nervous system
CO	Carbon monoxide
COPD	Chronic obstructive pulmonary disease
CPN	Community psychiatric nurse
CRP	C-reactive protein
CSF	Cerebrospinal fluid
CSU	Catheter stream urine sample
CT	Computerised tomography

CTPA	Computerised tomography pulmonary angiogram
CVA	Cerebrovascular accident
CVP	Central venous pressure
CXR	Chest X-ray
DC	Direct current
DIC	Disseminated intravascular coagulation
DKA	Diabetic ketoacidosis
DMARD	Disease-modifying anti-rheumatic drugs
DNACPR	Do not attempt cardiopulmonary resuscitation
DNAR	Do not attempt resuscitation
DNR	Do not resuscitate
DOAC	Direct oral anticoagulant
Dr	Doctor
dsDNA	Double-stranded DNA (antibodies)
DSM	Diagnostic and Statistical Manual of Mental Disorders
DVLA	Driver and Vehicle Licensing Agency
DVT	Deep vein thrombosis
Dx	Diagnosis
DXA	Dual-energy X-ray absorptiometry
EBV	Epstein–Barr virus
ECG	Electrocardiogram
ED	Emergency department
EEG	Electroencephalogram
eGFR	Estimated glomerular filtration rate
EMU	Early morning urine sample
ENA	Extractable nuclear antigen
ERCP	Endoscopic retrograde cholangiopancreatography
ESR	Erythrocyte sedimentation rate
ESRF	End-stage renal failure
EUA	Examination under anaesthetic
FBC	Full blood count
FiO$_2$	Fraction of inspired oxygen
FLAIR	Fluid attenuation inversion recovery
FSH	Follicle-stimulating hormone
FY1 FY2	Foundation Doctor [year 1 or year 2]
GA	General anaesthetic
GBM	Glomerular basement membrane
GBS	Guillain–Barré syndrome
GCA	Giant cell arteritis
GCS	Glasgow Coma Score
G-CSF	Granulocyte colony-stimulating factor
GFR	Glomerular filtration rate
GI	Gastrointestinal
GMC	General Medical Council
GORD	Gastro-oesophageal reflux disease
GP	General Practitioner
h/o	History of
HACEK	Haemophilus species, Aggregatibacter species, Cardiobacterium species, *Eikenella corrodens*, Kingella species
Hb	Haemoglobin
HbA1c	Haemoglobin A1c
HCA	Healthcare assistant
HCSW	Healthcare support worker
HDL	High-density lipoprotein
HDU	High Dependency Unit
HELLP	Haemolysis, elevated liver enzymes, low platelet count
HHS	Hyperglycaemic hyperosmolar state
HIT	Heparin-induced thrombocytopenia
HIV	Human immunodeficiency virus
HRS	Hepatorenal syndrome
HRT	Hormone replacement therapy
HSV	Herpes simplex virus

Ht	Height		**LH**	Luteinising hormone
HUS	Haemolytic uraemic syndrome		**LMP**	Last menstrual period
Hx	History		**LMWH**	Low molecular weight heparin
i	One tablet		**LP**	Lumbar puncture
ii	Two tablets		**LTOT**	Long-term oxygen therapy
iii	Three tablets		**MC&S**	Microscopy, culture and sensitivities
i.m., IM	Injection into a muscle		**M/R**	Modified release
i.v., IV	Injection directly to a vein		**MCA**	Middle cerebral artery
IBD	Inflammatory bowel disease		**MCP**	Metacarpophalangeal joint
IBS	Irritable bowel syndrome		**MCV**	Mean corpuscular volume
IECOPD	Infective exacerbation of COPD		**MDT**	Multidisciplinary Team
IgA	Immunoglobulin A		**MI**	Myocardial infarction
IgE	Immunoglobulin E		**MRC**	Medical Research Council
IGF-1	Insulin-like growth factor-1		**MRCP**	Magnetic resonance cholangiopancreatography
IgG	Immunoglobulin G			
IgM	Immunoglobulin M		**MRI**	Magnetic resonance imaging
ILD	Interstitial lung disease		**MRSA**	Methicillin-resistant *Staphylococcus aureus*
INR	International normalised ratio			
IPF	Idiopathic pulmonary fibrosis		**MS**	Multiple sclerosis
ITP	Immune thrombocytopenic purpura		**MSU**	Mid-stream urine sample
ITU	Intensive Therapy Unit or Intensive Care Unit		**MV**	Mitral valve
			NaCl	Sodium chloride
IV	Intravenous		**NAD**	No abnormality detected
IVI	Intravenous infusion		**NAI**	Non-accidental injury
Ix	Investigations		**NBM**	Nil by mouth
JVP	Jugular venous pressure		**NEWS**	National Early Warning Score
KUB	Kidney, ureters, bladder		**NG**	Nasogastric
LA	Local anaesthetic		**NHS**	National Health Service
LABA	Long-acting beta-2 agonist		**NICE**	National Institute for Health and Care Excellence
LAMA	Long-acting muscarinic agonist			
LDH	Lactate dehydrogenase		**NIV**	Non-invasive ventilation
LDL	Low-density lipoprotein		**NOAC**	Novel oral anticoagulant
LFT	Liver function test		**NOCTE**	Every night
			NoF	Neck of femur

NSAID	Nonsteroidal anti-inflammatory drug		**PTT**	Partial thromboplastin time
NSTEMI	Non-ST elevation myocardial infarction		**PV**	Pulmonary valve
o.d., od, OD	Once a day		**q.d.s., qds., QDS**	Four times a day
o/e	On examination		**RCC**	Red cell count
OA	Osteoarthritis		**ROSC**	Return of spontaneous circulation
OGD	Oesophagogastroduodenoscopy		**RRT**	Renal replacement therapy
OT	Occupational Therapist		**RSI**	Repetitive strain injuries
p.c.	After food		**RTA**	Road traffic accident
p.m., pm, PM	Afternoon or evening		**Rx**	Treatment
p.o., po, PO	Orally / by mouth / oral administration		**s.c., SC**	Injection under the skin
p.r., pr, PR	Rectally		**S/R**	Sustained release
p.r.n., prn, PRN	As needed		**SAH**	Subarachnoid haemorrhage
p/c	Presenting complaint		**SBP**	Spontaneous bacterial peritonitis
PA	Postero-anterior		**SLE**	Systemic lupus erythematosus
PaCO$_2$	Partial pressure of carbon dioxide		**SLICC**	Systemic Lupus Erythematosus International Collaborating Clinics
PaO$_2$	Partial pressure of oxygen		**SLT**	Speech and Language Therapist
PBC	Primary biliary cirrhosis or Primary biliary cholangitis		**SOL**	Space-occupying lesion
PCI	Percutaneous coronary intervention		**SpR**	Specialist registrar
PCR	Polymerase chain reaction		**SSRI**	Selective serotonin reuptake inhibitor
PE	Pulmonary embolism or pulmonary embolus		**stat.**	Immediately, with no delay, now
PEG	Percutaneous endoscopic gastrostomy		**STEMI**	ST-elevation myocardial infarction
physio	Physiotherapist		**t.d.s., tds., TDS**	Three times a day
PIP	Proximal interphalangeal joint		**TAVI**	Transcatheter aortic valve implantation
POP	Plaster of Paris		**TB**	Tuberculosis
PPCM	Peripartum cardiomyopathy		**TFT**	Thyroid function test
PSC	Primary sclerosing cholangitis		**TNF**	Tumour necrosis factor
PT	Prothrombin time		**TPMT**	Thiopurine methyltransferase
PTH	Parathyroid hormone		**TPN**	Total parenteral nutrition
			TRH	Thyrotropin-releasing hormone
			TSH	Thyroid-stimulating hormone

TTP	Thrombotic thrombocytopenic purpura	**VEGF**	Vascular endothelial growth factor
TV	Tricuspid valve	**Vit**	Vitamin
U&E	Urea and electrolytes	**VSD**	Ventricular septal defect
UC	Ulcerative colitis	**WCC**	White cell count
UGIB	Upper gastrointestinal bleed	**WE**	Wernicke encephalopathy
UTI	Urinary tract infection	**WHO**	World Health Organization
VATS	Video-assisted thoracoscopic surgery		

Index

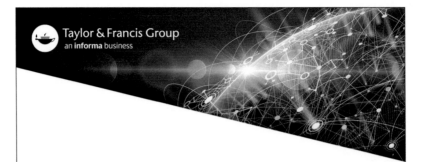